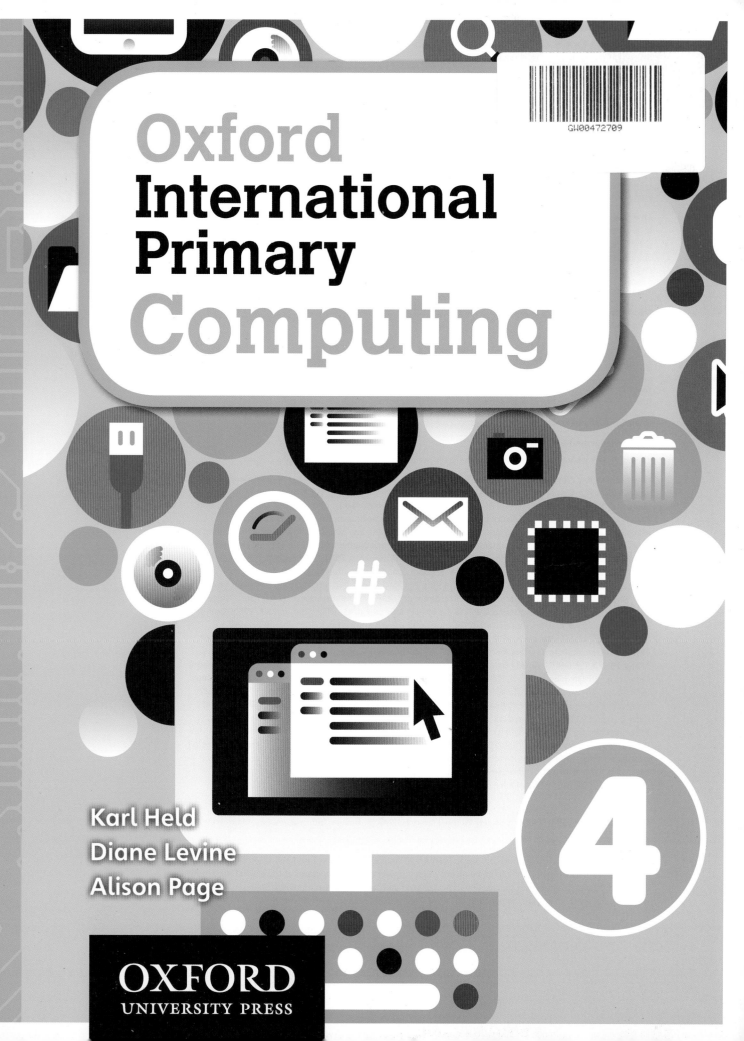

Oxford
International Primary
Computing

Karl Held
Diane Levine
Alison Page

4

OXFORD
UNIVERSITY PRESS

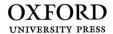

1.99 (14)

Great Clarendon Street, Oxford, OX2 6DP, United Kingdom

Oxford University Press is a department of the University of Oxford. It furthers the University's objective of excellence in research, scholarship, and education by publishing worldwide. Oxford is a registered trade mark of Oxford University Press in the UK and in certain other countries

British Library Cataloguing in Publication Data
Data available

978-0-19-831000-6

3 5 7 9 10 8 6 4 2

Paper used in the production of this book is a natural, recyclable product made from wood grown in sustainable forests. The manufacturing process conforms to the environmental regulations of the country of origin.

Printed in China by Printplus Ltd

Acknowledgements

The publishers would like to thank the following for permissions to use their photographs:

Cover illustration: Alberto Antoniazzi, P4-5: John M Anderson/Shutterstock, P6: iStock.com, P7a: Elena Schweitzer/ Shutterstock, P7b: Zocchi Roberto/Shutterstock, P8: Image Source/Corbis, P13: iStock.com, P14a: Wet nose/ Shutterstock, P14b: Shutterstock, P20-21a: 123rf, P20b: Image Source / Alamy, P21: Radub85/ Dreamstime.com, P22a: Science & Society Picture Library /SSPL/Getty Images, P22b: iStock.com, P22c: Informat /Alamy, P22d: Shutterstock, P23a: Iakov Kalinin/Shutterstock, P23b: f4foto/Alamy, P24: JHPhoto /Alamy, P26a: Shutterstock, P26b: Puwadol Jaturawutthichai/ Shutterstock, P27a: Joshua Resnick/Shutterstock, P27b: Michael Hurcomb/ Corbis, P28a: iStock.com, P28b: Dreamstime.com, P28c: Dreamstime.com, P28d: Shutterstock, P33: Shutterstock, P34: Alya Ivanova/ Moment Open/Getty Images, P36: iStock.com, P37a: Shutterstock, P37b: iStock.com, P37c: iStock.com, P37d: iStock.com, P38: Galya Ivanova, P40: iStock.com, P42: Shutterstock, P48: Shutterstock, P51: Vibe Images /Alamy, P52a: Shutterstock, P52b: Shutterstock, P53: Vladimir Arkatov/123rf, P56a: Shutterstock, P56b: Shutterstock, P68-69: Shutterstock, P71: Ryan Bird, P73: Shutterstock, P75a: Shutterstock, P75b: Andrey Starostin/Shutterstock, P75c: Shutterstock, P76: Pratchaya Ruenyen/Shutterstock, P78: Catalin Petolea/ Shutterstock, P79a: Shutterstock, P79b: Shutterstock, P80: Shutterstock, P81a: Georgios Kollidas/Shutterstock, P81b: Shutterstock, P81c: Piti Tan/Shutterstock, P83: M. Unal Ozmen/Shutterstock, P84-85: ZUMA Press, Inc. / Alamy, P85: OUISA GOULIAMAKI / Stringer/ AFP/Getty Images, P86: Jean-Pierre Lescourret/ Lonely Planet Images/ Getty Images, P88a: John Eskenazi, P88b: Leslie Garland Picture Library /Alamy, P90a: Melvyn Longhurst /Alamy, P90b: Rasoul ali / Moment/Getty Images, P90c: Public Domain, P92a: Library of Congress/Science Faction/ Getty Images, P92b: Science & Society Picture Library /SSPL /Getty Images, P92c: Michael Melford/ The Image Bank/ Getty Images, P92d: Pictorial Press Ltd / Alamy, P93: Microstockeurope / Alamy, P94a: Science Photo Library, P94b: Bletchley Park Trust / SSPL/Getty Images, P94c: Patrick AVENTURIER / Gamma-Rapho/Getty Images, P95: Mark Williamson/Science Photo Library, P96a: Sam Ogden/Science Photo Library, P96b: Thomas Jurkowski / Dreamstime.com, P98a: Library of Congress/Science Faction/ Getty Images, P98b: Melvyn Longhurst / Alamy, P98c: John Eskenazi, P98d: Science Photo Library, P98e: Pictorial Press Ltd / Alamy, P99a: Public Domain, P99b:Thomas Jurkowski / Dreamstime.com, P99c: Science & Society Picture Library /SSPL /Getty Images

Workbook:

LESSON 2.1, left to right: Science & Society Picture Library /SSPL/Getty Images, Informat / Alamy, Shutterstock

Lesson 2.5: Shutterstock

Although we have made every effort to trace and contact all copyright holders before publication this has not been possible in all cases. If notified, the publisher will rectify any errors or omissions at the earliest opportunity. Links to third party websites are provided by Oxford in good faith and for information only. Oxford disclaims any responsibility for the materials contained in any third party website referenced in this work.

Contents

1 Working with text: Are you hungry?

By the end of this unit you will know:

→ how to plan the layout of a page

→ how to align your words

→ how to store your files

→ how to cut, copy and paste text

→ how to find and replace text in a long document

→ how to give feedback to someone else.

In this unit you are going to make a set of recipes for a food website.

The internet has changed the way we cook. We can use it to find out lots of information about different types of food and the way food affects our bodies. We can also share recipes.

Activity Favourite foods

What is your favourite meal? Can you make a list of the ingredients?

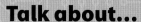

Talk about...

Why do you like your favourite meal so much? What does it taste like? Does it make you think of special people, places or times? What does it look like?

align   cut   copy
file   document
feedback   hierarchical
find and replace   shared
paste

Fascinating fact

There are more than 2,000 different types of plant that humans grow for food.

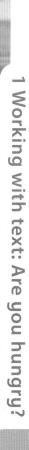

You will remember:

→ how to open a new file
→ how to open a file that already exists
→ important keys on the keyboard
→ how to find your way around the toolbar
→ how to save a file.

You already know how to do quite a lot of important things on the computer. Let's see what you remember.

How to open and save files
Try doing all of these things:

1 Save a new file or save an updated file.

2 Open a file you have saved before.

3 Open a new **file**.

4 Find your way around the keyboard.

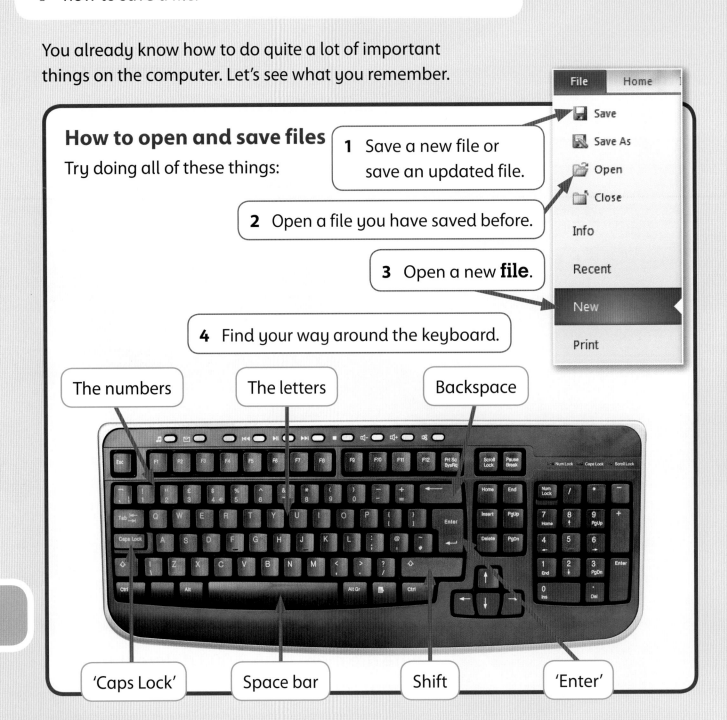

The numbers
The letters
Backspace
'Caps Lock'
Space bar
Shift
'Enter'

File   Home
- Save
- Save As
- Open
- Close
- Info
- Recent
- New
- Print

How to use the toolbar

What do you remember about the toolbar? What sorts of things can you do with it? Try one of these:

→ Insert an image.

→ Change the font size.

→ Change the font style.

→ Change the font colour.

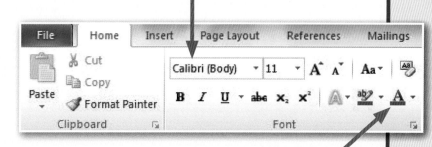

Do you remember what 'font' means?

An 'icon' is a small picture.

Activity Invent a new toolbar

1 Imagine that you have invented a new type of software program. It can do anything you like.

   → It could be for designing sweets.

   → It could be for designing a vegetable garden.

2 Imagine your software has a toolbar. What sorts of things will the toolbar do? What icons will you have?

3 Draw your toolbar.

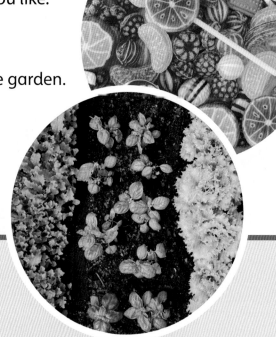

If you have time...

Share your toolbar with a friend.
Can your friend think of any more icons?

You will learn:

➔ how to align text on a page.

Talk about...

What do you notice about the way this recipe is laid out?

Home	Recipes	Blog	Store	ContactUs

Biscuits

Ingredients:

60 g plain flour

40 g butter (room temperature)

½ teaspoon vanilla extract

20 g caster sugar

Instructions:

1 Wash your hands.

2 Measure your ingredients.

3 Mix the flour and butter together in a mixing bowl.

4 Add the vanilla extract and sugar.

5 Squeeze the mixture until it sticks together.

6 Roll it out with a rolling pin.

7 Use a cutter to cut out biscuit shapes. Place them on a baking tray.

8 Bake in the oven at 160°C Fan/180°C/ Gas 3 for 12–15 minutes.

You will see that some of the words are **aligned** in the centre of the page. 'Align' means to position the text on the page.

Activity Plan a recipe layout

Use the worksheet your teacher has given you to plan your recipe.

Which words will you place in the centre of the page?

How to align text
Aligning text in a new document

Open a new **document**.

Click on the 'Center' icon. Then type a word or sentence. It will be in the middle of the page.

Press the 'Enter' key to start a new line.

Click on the 'Align Text Left' icon. Then type a word or sentence. It will be on the left of the page.

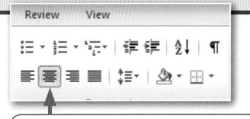

Click the 'Center' icon on the toolbar.

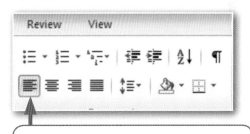

Click the 'Align Text Left' icon.

Aligning text in a document that you have been working on

You can also use these icons to align text in a document that already exists.

Highlight the text you want to centre. Click the 'Center' icon.

Highlight the text you want to left align. Click the 'Align Text Left' icon.

Activity Align text

Your teacher will give you a document called 'Biscuits recipe'.
You can see that it hasn't been aligned very well!
Your job is to improve the alignment.

1 Centre the title and the headings.

2 Left align the ingredients and the instructions.

You will learn:

→ how to store your files in a sensible way.

Sometimes we save files in folders that only we use.

But sometimes we do work in a group, and we all need to use a **shared** folder. Shared means something that a group of people can access or use.

Folders are **hierarchical**. That's a big word! It means that folders are organised in levels. You can create a shared folder in a hierarchy.

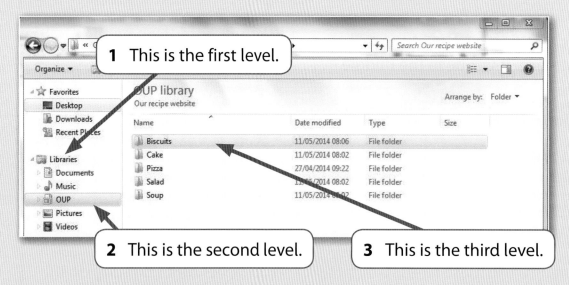

1 This is the first level.

2 This is the second level.

3 This is the third level.

How to create a shared folder

Sit in your group. Your teacher will show you where to put your shared folder.

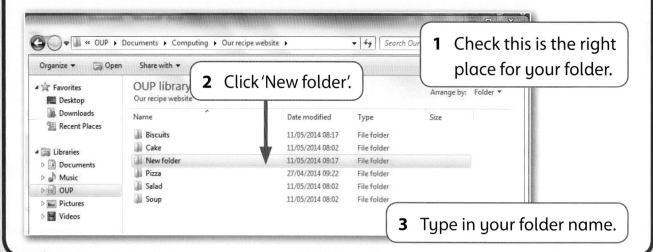

1 Check this is the right place for your folder.

2 Click 'New folder'.

3 Type in your folder name.

Activity Shared folders

1 Work with a group. Work together to invent a new recipe.

➔ You can use real ingredients or made-up ingredients such as moonlight or beetles.

➔ Your recipe can be sweet or savoury, sensible or silly.

➔ The recipe is for a website, not for a cookbook.

2 Create a shared folder that you can use to save your recipe.

3 Give the folder the name of your recipe.

4 Each person in the group should type one part of the recipe in a separate file. The jobs are to create:

➔ the layout

➔ the ingredients

➔ the equipment

➔ the instructions.

It does not matter if you do not finish your typing in this lesson.

5 Save your files in the shared folder at the end of the lesson. Give each file a name that tells you what it contains.

Talk about...

Why was it useful to work in a group?

You will learn:

→ how to cut, copy and paste text.

Sometimes we want to move words from one part of a document to another, or from one document to another.

We might want to **cut** the text

or we might want to **copy** the text.

We can then **paste** the text somewhere else.

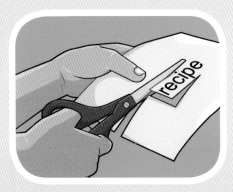 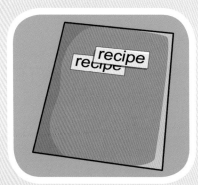 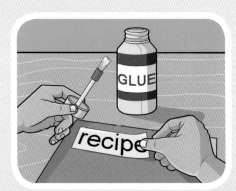

How to cut, copy and paste

There are two ways to cut, copy and paste. You can use the icons on the toolbar, or the keys on the keyboard.

1 Using the toolbar

Click the 'Home' tab on the toolbar.

Highlight the text you want to cut or copy.

Click where you want the text to go.

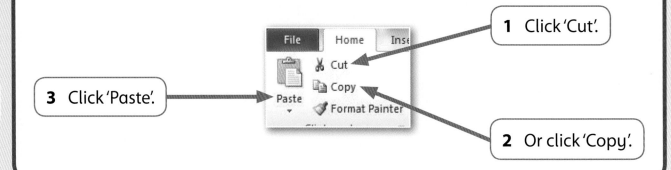

1 Click 'Cut'.

3 Click 'Paste'.

2 Or click 'Copy'.

2 Using the keyboard

Highlight the text you want to cut, copy or paste.

Press and hold the 'Ctrl' key and press the 'C' key to copy.

Press and hold the 'Ctrl' key and press the 'X' key to cut.

Click where you want the text to go.

Press and hold the 'Ctrl' key and press the 'V' key to paste.

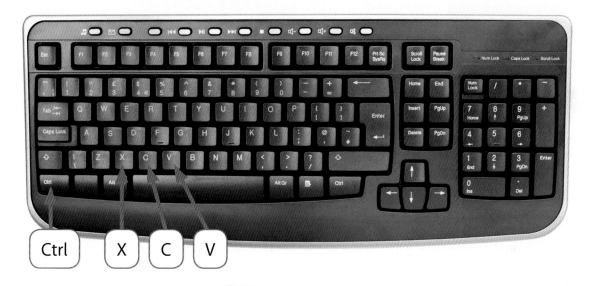

Ctrl   X   C   V

Activity   Bringing it all together

1 Open your shared folder. Open the layout file and the ingredients file.

2 Highlight the text in the ingredients file. Copy or cut the text you want to move to the shared file.

3 Go to the layout file. Click where you want the text to go.

4 Paste in the text.

5 Do this for the rest of the recipe.

If you have time...

You can use copy, cut and paste to move text around inside a document. Rearrange the order of the text in your recipe file until you are happy with how it looks.

Talk about...

When is it useful to copy and paste?

13

You will learn:

→ how to find words in a document
→ how to replace words in a document.

Some documents are short like this poster.

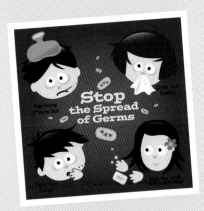

Other documents are long like this book.

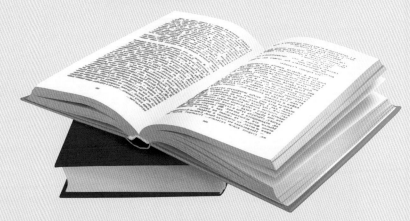

You can use a command called **find and replace** to find a word in a document. You might want to change a word throughout the document. For example, you might want to change 'butter' to 'margarine'. Find and replace will save you time and you won't miss any words.

How to find and replace a word

Look at the toolbar.

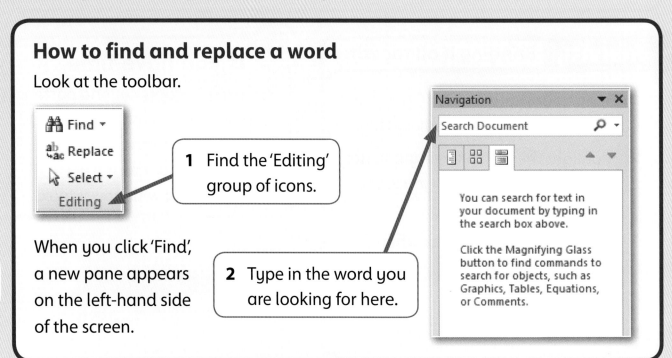

1 Find the 'Editing' group of icons.

When you click 'Find', a new pane appears on the left-hand side of the screen.

2 Type in the word you are looking for here.

You can search for text in your document by typing in the search box above.

Click the Magnifying Glass button to find commands to search for objects, such as Graphics, Tables, Equations, or Comments.

When you click 'Replace', a new dialog box opens.

1 Type in the word you are looking for here.

2 Type in the word you want to replace it with here.

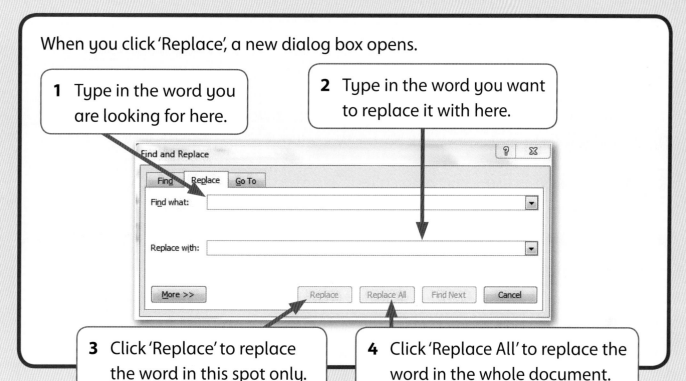

3 Click 'Replace' to replace the word in this spot only.

4 Click 'Replace All' to replace the word in the whole document.

Activity | Find and replace

1 Open your recipe file.

2 Choose an ingredient. Think of something else you could use instead.

3 Use the find and replace command to find all the examples of the word in your recipe.

4 Replace it with your new ingredient.

If you are not happy with the change you have made, you can use the find and replace command to change it back again.

Activity | Finish your recipe

Look again at your recipe. Do you need to complete any more work on it?

 If you have time…

You can use the keyboard to find words instead of the toolbar. Press and hold the 'Ctrl' and 'F' keys together. What happens?

You will learn:

➔ how to give helpful feedback.

It is sometimes helpful to have someone else look at work we have done. They can help us to make the work better. We call this giving **feedback**.

 We are going to use something called 'Two Stars and a Wish' to give feedback to our classmates in this lesson.

How to give constructive feedback

'Two Stars and a Wish' helps us to focus on improving the work. This way we are less likely to hurt someone else's feelings. Here is an example.

Fruit sundae

Ingredients:
Strawberries or any fruit you like
5 tablespoons oats
2 tablespoons honey
8 tablespoons yoghurt
A tall glass

Instructions:
1. Mix the oats and the honey.
2. Put them in the bottom of your glass.
3. Pour the yoghurt on top of the oats.
4. Fill the rest of the glass with strawberries or any other fruit you like.

Two Stars and a Wish

Name of recipe:	Fruit sundae
★	I especially like the recipe title. It is bold and a different colour so it stands out.
★	I can see that you have checked the spelling. There are no spelling mistakes in the recipe.
	I wish you would use bold text for the headings Ingredients and Instructions.

Here are some other things to remember when you are giving your feedback:

➔ Only talk about this piece of work. Avoid using phrases like 'you always'.

➔ Say how the work made you feel. You could use a sentence like, 'It made me feel interested when I saw the…' or 'I felt bored when I saw the…'.

➔ Try to be very clear when you are making a suggestion to improve the work. For example, you could say 'I wish you would add an interesting font style to your heading', rather than 'I wish you would make it look nicer.'

Activity | Two stars and a wish

1 Open your group's recipe file.

2 Print a copy of your recipe.

3 Share it with another group.

4 Look at their recipe while they look at yours.

   ➔ Have they checked it has correct grammar and spelling?

   ➔ Have they used font size, colour or style to make any words look special?

   ➔ Is their text aligned in a way that will look good on a website?

   ➔ Will the recipe look good on a website?

5 Find two things that the group has done well. You will give them a star for these two things.

6 Find one thing that you 'wish' the group had done differently.

7 Complete the 'Two Stars and a Wish' feedback form and give it to the other group.

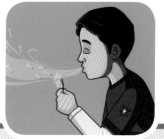

 If you have time…

Make changes to your recipe based on the feedback you have received.

What you have learned about working with text

In this unit you have learned:

→ how to plan the layout of a page

→ how to align text on a page

→ how to find words in a document

→ how to replace words in a document

→ how to cut, copy and paste text

→ how to store your files in a sensible way

→ how to give helpful feedback.

1 Match the command with the keyboard keys.

1	Copy	**a**	Ctrl X
2	Paste	**b**	Ctrl F
3	Cut	**c**	Ctrl C
4	Find	**d**	Ctrl V

2 Which of these icons would you choose to align text in the middle of a page?

a   b   c   d

_____

3 Which of these icons would you choose to align text on the left of the page?

a   b   c   d

_____

18

Activity Give feedback on a recipe

Your teacher will show you a recipe from a food website. Find 'Two Stars and a Wish' for the page.

  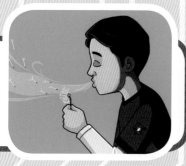

Activity Improve this document

 1 Your teacher will give you a recipe. Can you make these changes to make it look better?

   a Align some text.

   b Find the word **strawberries**. How many times does it appear in the recipe?

   c Change the size or colour of the title.

2 Now make a new folder. Save the document into the new folder.

> Strawberry and yoghurt ice lollies
>
> Ingredients:
> 250 g strawberries
> 100 g yoghurt
> 1 teaspoon honey
>
> Equipment:
> a bowl
> a fork
> 4 ice lolly moulds
> 4 lolly sticks
>
> Instructions:
> 1. Put the strawberries in a bowl.
> 2. Mash the strawberries with a fork.
> 3. Mix together the strawberries, yoghurt and honey.
> 4. Put the mixture into 4 ice lolly moulds.
> 5. Put a lolly stick into each mould.
> 6. Put the ice lollies in the freezer for at least 4 hours.

2 Multimedia: Photos for our recipes

By the end of this unit you will know:

→ how to plan a photo shoot for a project

→ how to take good photos using a digital camera

→ how to improve your photos using a computer

→ how to combine photos in a document to create an illustration to go with your text.

In this unit you are going to make, edit and combine digital photographs to illustrate a recipe.

Fascinating fact

The first photograph was made in 1826. Today, about 380 billion photographs are taken around the world every year. That's over 1 billion photographs every day.

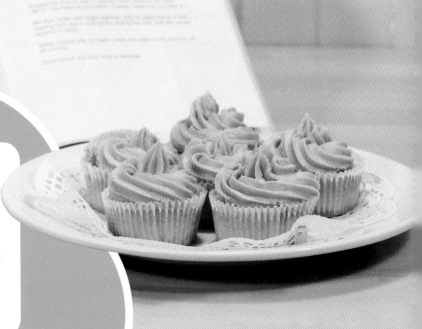

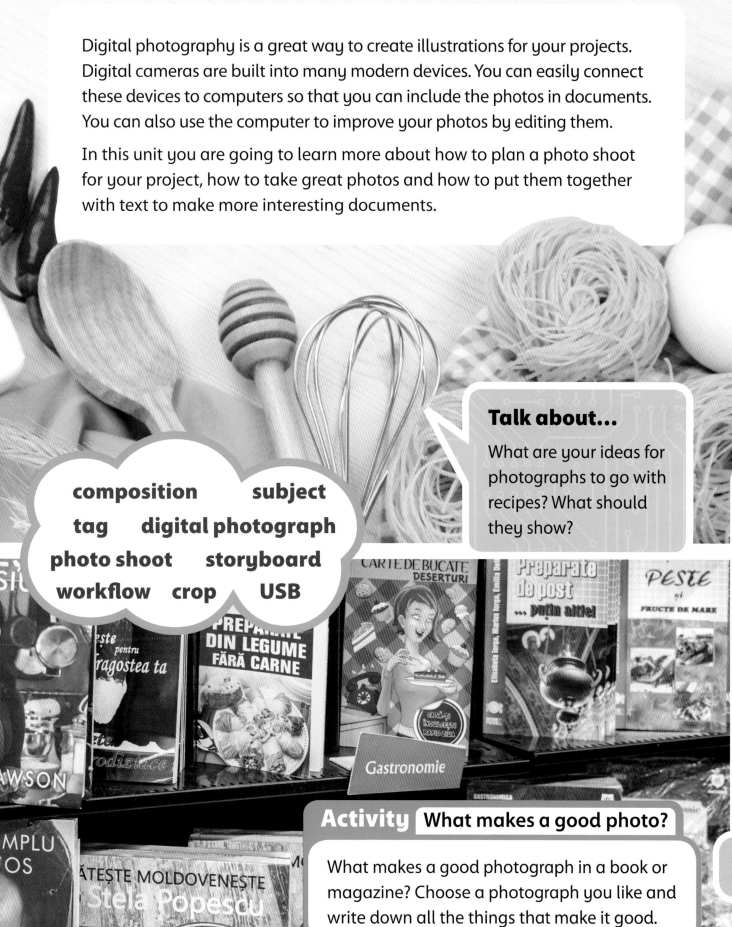

Digital photography is a great way to create illustrations for your projects. Digital cameras are built into many modern devices. You can easily connect these devices to computers so that you can include the photos in documents. You can also use the computer to improve your photos by editing them.

In this unit you are going to learn more about how to plan a photo shoot for your project, how to take great photos and how to put them together with text to make more interesting documents.

composition   subject
tag   digital photograph
photo shoot   storyboard
workflow   crop   USB

Talk about...

What are your ideas for photographs to go with recipes? What should they show?

Activity **What makes a good photo?**

What makes a good photograph in a book or magazine? Choose a photograph you like and write down all the things that make it good.

You will learn:

→ how photography has changed through history
→ how digital cameras help us take photos
→ that people use computers to store photographs
→ that people use computers to change photographs.

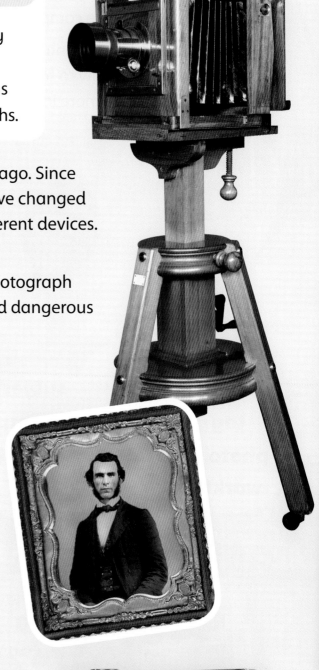

The first photographs were made about 200 years ago. Since then the cameras we use to make photographs have changed a lot. Nowadays, cameras are built in to many different devices.

Plate

The first cameras that could make a permanent photograph used a metal plate. The Daguerreotype process used dangerous chemicals such as mercury.

Film

The first cameras to use film were invented over 100 years ago. The 'Brownie' was the first cheap and easy to use camera in the world. Now anyone could be a photographer.

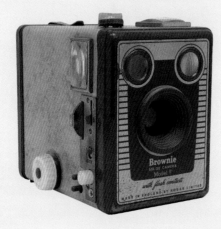

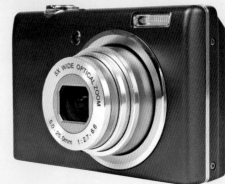

Digital

The technology to make **digital photographs** was available in the 1970s. In the 1990s digital cameras became reliable and cheap enough for most people. For the last 20 years, digital cameras have been more popular than film cameras.

Devices with built-in cameras

Digital cameras are now also built in to many other devices. For example, most smartphones have a built-in digital camera.

Cameras and computers

Digital cameras work together with computers. The cameras store photos as files. You can then use the computer to store and change images.

We can use picture editing software to:

→ crop photos

→ improve the brightness of a photo

→ remove red-eye reflections caused by a flash.

Professional designers sometimes change photographs so they look very different. This is often called 'photoshopping' because *Photoshop* is the name of the software that is used.

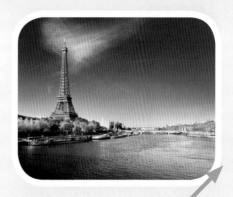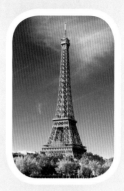

The shape of this photo has been changed. This is called 'cropping'.

The designer has changed the background colour.

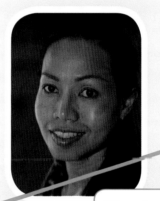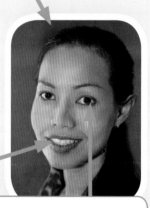

The designer has brightened the model's teeth.

The designer has removed the red-eye reflections.

Activity | Different types of camera

 On the worksheet write down three things about each of the cameras.

Write about how easy they are to use and how easy they are to carry. Why might they be designed like this?

If you have time...

On the worksheet write down the names of three devices that have digital cameras built in. Write down why each device has a camera.

You will learn:

→ how to plan a photo shoot for a recipe page.

When you are making photographs for a special purpose it helps to plan ahead. When professional photographers take photos for a project they call it a **photo shoot**. They always plan a photo shoot carefully so that they get all the right photographs for the project.

How to get ideas for your photo shoot

A good way to start planning a photo shoot is to look at how other people have used photographs to illustrate their work.

For your recipe photo shoot you could look at:

→ recipe books at school or at home

→ recipe websites and food blogs on the internet.

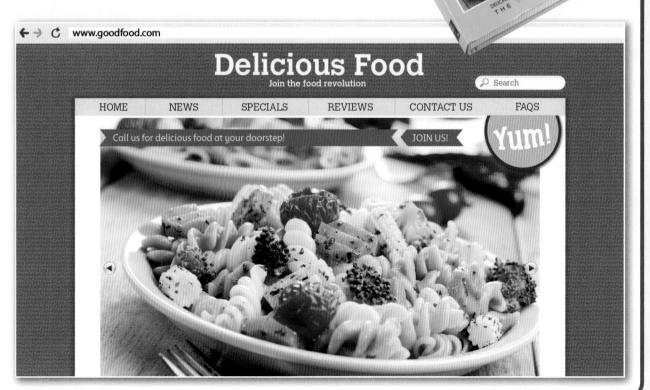

How to make a plan

Think about your recipe.

➜ What steps are there in the recipe? Which are the most important steps?

➜ Which steps will make the best photographs?

Think of your photos as telling a story. You don't have to have a photo for every part of the story – only the best bits. The photos should work together with the text to tell the story.

You can use a **storyboard** to help you decide what photos to include. A storyboard is a simple drawing that shows the order of the photos to tell the story. It also shows what should be in each photo.

For your recipe photo shoot the storyboard will help you decide what ingredients, equipment and actions should be in the photos.

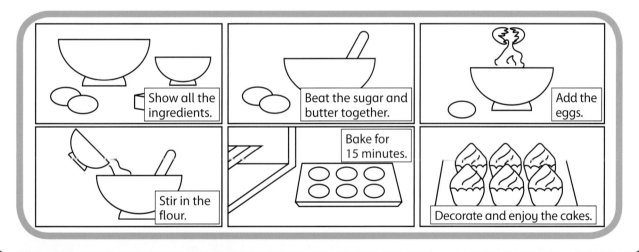

Show all the ingredients.

Beat the sugar and butter together.

Add the eggs.

Stir in the flour.

Bake for 15 minutes.

Decorate and enjoy the cakes.

Activity Plan a photo shoot

1 ⬇ On the worksheet, circle each step of the recipe that will make a good photograph. Write down why you think so.

2 ⬇ Use the template to draw a storyboard showing each of the steps you have chosen.

Talk about...

Discuss your choices for the recipe photos with your classmates. Do you all agree?

You will learn:

→ how to use a digital camera to make photographs
→ the three things to think about when you are taking a photograph.

You can use a digital camera or a smartphone to make great photographs. You will make better photographs if you remember a few simple rules.

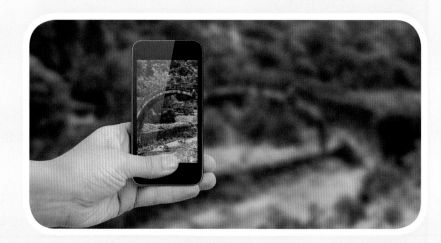

How to make good photographs

Composition

Every photograph has a **subject**. The subject is the main thing you want to show. You can decide where in your photo to place your subject. This is called **composition**.

In many photos the subject is in the centre of the picture. But you can put your subject in other places to make a more interesting composition.

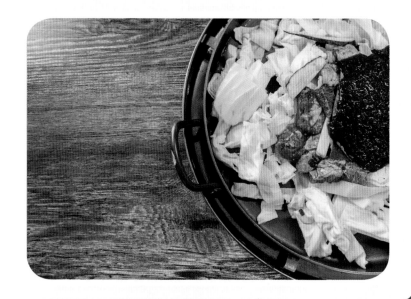

Decide how close you want to get to the subject. You can use the camera's zoom or just your own two feet to get closer.

Focus

You need to make sure the subject of your photo is in focus. This means that it looks clear and not blurred. Don't get too close. Many cameras can only focus on subjects that are further than 20 cm away.

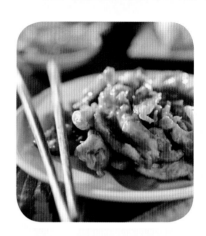

If your camera is focusing on the wrong part of the picture, you can move the camera slightly.

Lighting

Your camera can measure and control the amount of light that makes each photo. If there is too much light, the camera adjusts. If there is not enough light, the camera can use a flash to add more light.

You can use the screen of your camera to judge if there is enough light.

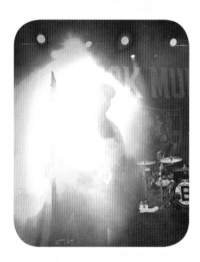

If the image on the screen looks very dark or if there are lots of coloured speckles (often called 'noise'), then there is probably not enough light to make a good photograph. You'll need to add some light or use the built-in flash.

◀ Using the flash is not always the best way. It can make the photo overexposed – this is when the edges of your photo are dark and the centre is too bright. This usually happens with close-up photos.

Activity Take photographs

1   Use the cameras and devices in class to take photographs of the subjects your teacher shows you.

2   Try different compositions: close-ups as well as distant shots.

Talk about...

Share your photos with your classmates and discuss them. Which look the best? And why?

You will learn:

→ connect your digital camera to copy photographs to a computer
→ use folders and tags to organise your photographs.

If you want to use your photos in a document or other project, you must transfer them from your digital camera or phone.

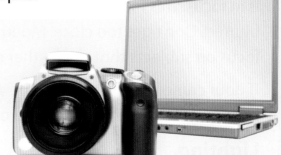

How to copy photographs to your computer

You can use a **USB** cable to connect most digital devices to your computer. There are different sizes of USB plug, called micro-, mini- and standard USB.

Insert the correct plug into your device and your computer.

Switch on your device. You will see the 'Autoplay' dialogue box.

> Click on 'Import pictures and videos using Windows Live Photo Gallery'.

You can add a description, called a **tag**, to help you remember important information about the pictures you are transferring.

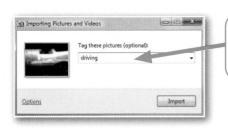

> Type your tag in the box.

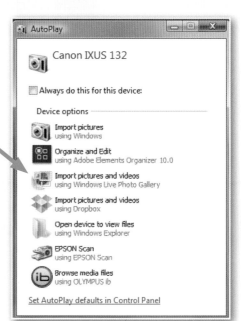

When you click 'OK' the computer will copy your photos from the device to the 'Pictures' folder on your computer.

How to organise photos on the computer

The photos will be stored in their own sub-folder. This folder will have the date and your tag in its name, for example: '2014-04-11 Recipe'.

You can view your photos in the 'Pictures Library' or 'Windows Live Photo Gallery'. You can also add tags to individual photos.

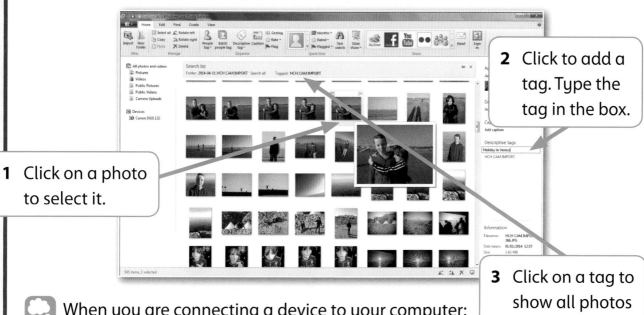

2 Click to add a tag. Type the tag in the box.

1 Click on a photo to select it.

3 Click on a tag to show all photos with that tag.

💭 When you are connecting a device to your computer:

→ Always ask permission from the device's owner.

→ Always ask permission from the computer's owner.

Activity | Transfer your photos

1 Connect your camera or other device to your computer and transfer your photos to the computer.

2 In the 'Picture Library' or 'Windows Live Photo Gallery', choose the photos you want to work on for your recipe.

3 Give each of these photos the same tag to help you find them again later.

Talk about...

Why do you need to ask permission before you connect a device to a computer?

You will learn how to:

→ improve your digital photos using a computer.

Sometimes photos from a digital camera are not perfect. You can use picture editing software on your computer to improve the exposure, colour and shape of your photos.

1 Use the 'Fine Tune' button to show the adjustment options.

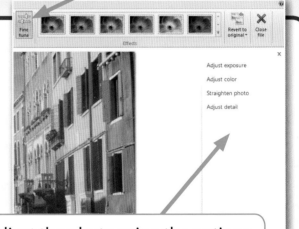

How to edit your photos

It is best to follow a proper order when you are editing your photos. This is called the **workflow**.

In *Windows Live Photo Gallery*, the 'Fine Tune' menu shows you the steps you should take.

1 Exposure

2 Adjust the photo using the options.

Always start with the 'Adjust exposure' settings. If the photo is too dark or too bright, you can change the brightness.

Move the 'Brightness' slider slowly to find the best position. The photo should be bright, but you should be able to see some detail in the lightest parts of the photo.

Next use the 'Contrast' slider to change the difference between the lightest and darkest areas. Move this slider slowly – you will see big changes in your photo. A colour photo changes very quickly from washed-out grey to very warm colours.

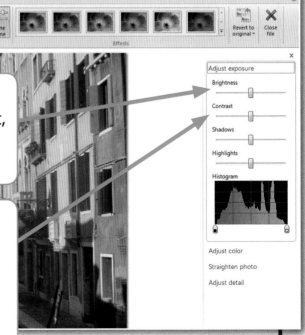

2 Colour

Next work on the colour settings.

> Use the 'Color temperature' slider. If you move the slider to the left, the photo becomes more blue and feels 'cooler'. If you move it to the right, the photo becomes more red and feels 'warmer'.

> The 'Saturation' slider controls how strongly the colours appear in the image. If you move it all the way to the left, you'll create a black and white image.

3 Composition

Finally, you can **crop** your photo to improve the composition.

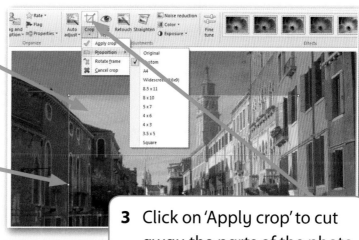

> **1** Click in the box to move it around the image.

> **2** Drag the handles to resize the box.

> **3** Click on 'Apply crop' to cut away the parts of the photo that are outside the box.

Activity Edit a photograph

1 Open your photo and follow the instructions to improve it.

2 Use the exposure settings to improve the photo. Use the brightness and contrast sliders to find the best solution.

3 Use the colour settings to create a natural colour look.

4 Use the cropping tool to highlight the main subject in the image.

You will learn how to:

→ add your photos to a text document

→ arrange the photos so that they fit together well with your text.

Word processing programs let you put words and pictures together to make your work look more interesting.

How to put a photo together with text

You can use the 'Wrap Text' menu to change how the text will fit around the photo.

You can also move, resize and rotate the photo.

Use the handles to make the photo bigger or smaller. Use the corner handles to make sure your photo doesn't get stretched or squashed.

Choose how your text will wrap around your image.

Picture Border
Picture Effects
Picture Layout
Position
Wrap Text
Bring Forward
Send Backward
Selection Pane

In Line with Text
Square
Tight
Through
Top and Bottom
Behind Text
In Front of Text
Edit Wrap Points
More Layout Options...

eryone knows how important it is to eat

althy food.

t fast food

be very

npting.

ny of us

uld eat

re fresh fruit and vegetables.

e key is to ha

Click on your photo and drag it to a new place.

Use the rotation handle at the top of the photo. Turn the photo so it is at an angle to other things on the page.

How to group photos together

You can use the 'Arrange' functions on the 'Picture Tools' toolbar to layer photos and other images like 'Shapes' to make a collage.

Making a collage

Use the cursor to arrange photos so that they overlap. Now click on a photo and use the 'Bring Forward' and 'Send Backward' buttons to change which photo is at the front. You now have a stack of photos.

Grouping photos

Select the stack of images: hold the shift key as you click on the photos one by one. Then click the 'Group' button to make your stack into a single image.

> This photo is behind all the others.

> This photo is in front of the others.

> Use these buttons to change the order of images.

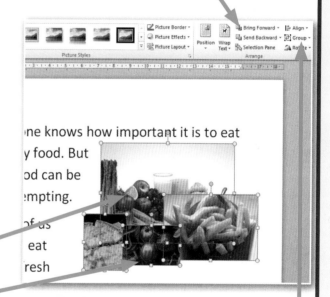

> Use the 'Group' button to make all the selected photos into one image.

Activity   Add photos to your recipe

1   Open your recipe document in *Microsoft Word*.

2   Insert the images you want to use to illustrate your recipe.

3   Move and resize the photos to create a layered collage.

4   Group the photos and place them with your recipe text on a single page.

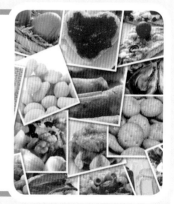

If you have time...

Use the 'Picture Styles' menu to add borders and effects to some of the photos.

What you have learned about multimedia

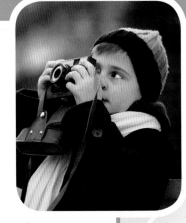

In this unit you have learned:

→ how to plan a photo shoot to make sure you get the photos you need for a project
→ how to take good photographs using a digital camera
→ how to improve your photos using a computer
→ how to combine photos in a document to create an illustration to go with your text.

The activities on this page will let you see how much you have learned.

1 What do these words mean?

composition

_____

_____

workflow

_____

_____

USB

_____

_____

2 What is the correct order of the steps in the picture editing workflow? Write these steps in the correct order.

_____

_____

_____

Adjust the colour.
Crop the photo.
Adjust the exposure.

34

Activity Storyboard

Draw a storyboard to plan a photo shoot for one of these events:

→ making a cup of coffee

→ launching a rocket to the moon.

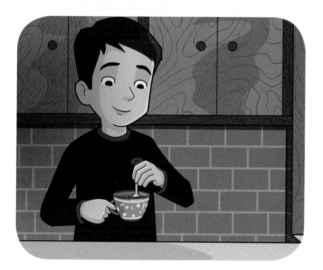

→ going to the cinema

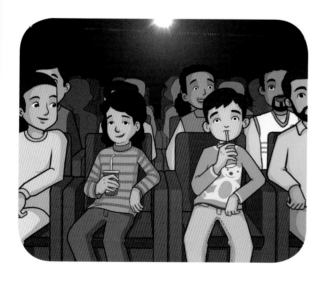

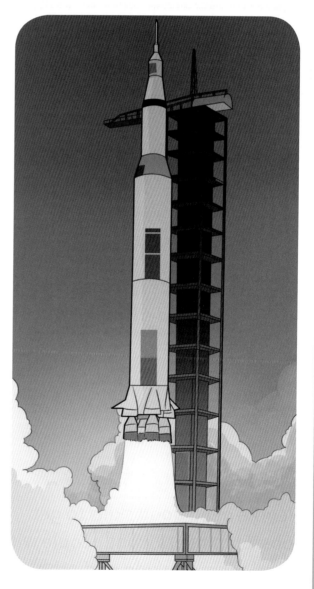

Include a maximum of six pictures in your storyboard. Write a caption for each picture in the storyboard. It should explain what the photo will show and why you have chosen it.

3 Handling data: Working with values

By the end of this unit you will know:

→ how to store number values using a spreadsheet

→ how to use spreadsheet functions

→ how to create spreadsheet formulas using cell references

→ how to make pie charts and bar charts that show your number values.

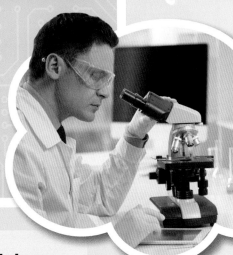

In this unit you are going to use a spreadsheet to calculate percentages and to make graphs.

Fascinating fact

People need good skills to get jobs. Employers want people with good team working and problem solving skills. They also want computer and number skills.

Which of these skills are you learning at school?

A spreadsheet is a type of computer software. It stores information and works out the answers to sums. The spreadsheet can draw graphs for you. In this unit you will do all of these things.

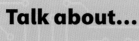

Talk about...

Make a class collection of job adverts from newspapers or the internet. Which of these jobs use computer skills?

Talk about your dream job with a friend. How will computers help you to do your dream job?

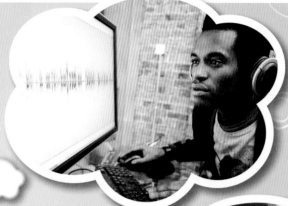

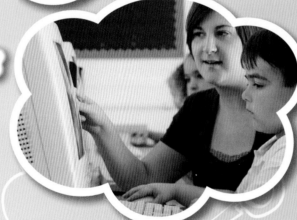

Activity | What do you want to be?

1 As a class, talk about what you want to be when you grow up. Your teacher will write a list of the most popular jobs.

2 Put a sticker next to the job that you like best.

3 Count how many stickers there are next to each job.

You can make a poster or a word-processed document with this information.

formula

bar chart   function

percentage   AutoSum

sum   cell reference

pie chart   segment

cell

You will learn:

→ what values and labels are
→ how to make a spreadsheet by entering values and labels into cells
→ how to format a spreadsheet.

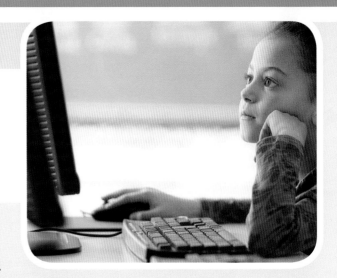

Cells and cell references

A spreadsheet is a grid of columns and rows.

Where a column crosses a row it makes a **cell**. The **cell reference** is the name of a cell. It is made of the column letter and the row number.

Values and labels

Spreadsheet cells can hold labels or values.

→ **Values** are numbers and calculations. Values are displayed on the right of the cell.

→ **Labels** are all other content, usually words. Labels are displayed on the left of a cell. If a label is too big it will spill into the cells next to it.

In this lesson you will make a spreadsheet with data about what students want to be when they grow up.

> The label in cell A1 is the heading for the spreadsheet.

How to put data into a spreadsheet

→ Select a cell with the cursor.

→ Click on the cell.

→ Enter a label. Press the 'Enter' key.

Repeat this to enter all the labels for your spreadsheet.

> This is the list of jobs. Each job label is in a different cell.

	A	B	C	D	E
1	Class survey				
2					
3	What do you want to be when you grow up?				
4					
5	Doctor				
6	Computer programmer				
7	Business person				
8	Home-maker and parent				
9	Singer or actor				
10	Teacher				
11	Something else				

A18

How to make the spreadsheet look better

You can:

➔ format the heading to stand out from the other labels

➔ make column A wider so it is big enough for all the labels.

1 Click and drag the line between column A and column B to make this column wider.

2 Use text formatting tools to format cells.

When you move the cursor to the line between columns A and B, it will change to this shape.

3 Make the heading larger and bolder than the other labels.

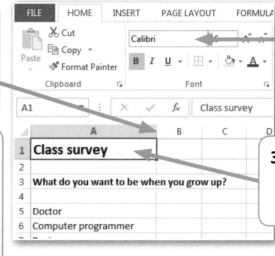

Activity Create a spreadsheet

1 Create a spreadsheet with a list of jobs.

2 In the next column enter the number of students who chose each job.

3 Use the text formatting tools to make the spreadsheet look better.

	A	B	C
1	**Class survey**		
2			
3	**What do you want to be when you grow up?**		
4			
5	Doctor	4	
6	Computer programmer	2	
7	Business person	7	
8	Home-maker and parent	3	
9	Singer or actor	6	
10	Teacher	5	

Talk about...

Look at the top of the spreadsheet screen and at the top of a word processing screen. Which things are the same? Why do you think they are the same? How does that help you use this software?

You will learn:

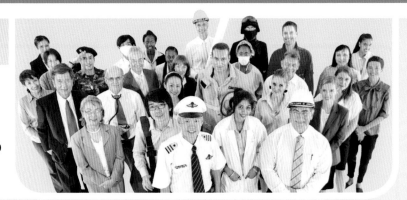

→ what a spreadsheet function is
→ what 'sum' means
→ how to use the Sum function to add up a column of numbers.

We often use the word 'sums' to mean any maths calculations. But when we are talking about maths or spreadsheets, the word **sum** means to add up a list of values.

The mathematical symbol for sum is the Greek letter Sigma: $\sum$

A spreadsheet **function** is a command that uses values in your spreadsheet to make a new value. Sum is a spreadsheet function.

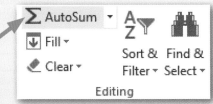

The **AutoSum** button lets you add 'Sum' to your spreadsheet.

How to use the Sum function

You will use the spreadsheet function 'Sum' to add up the total for your spreadsheet.

1 Enter the label 'Total'.

2 Select the cell where you want the total to appear.

3 Click on 'AutoSum'.

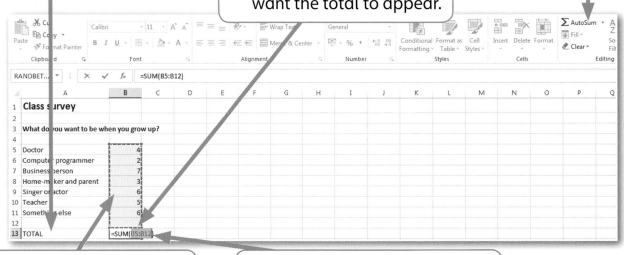

4 The computer will add together all the numbers in these cells.

5 B5:B12 means the computer will add together all the cells from B5 to B12.

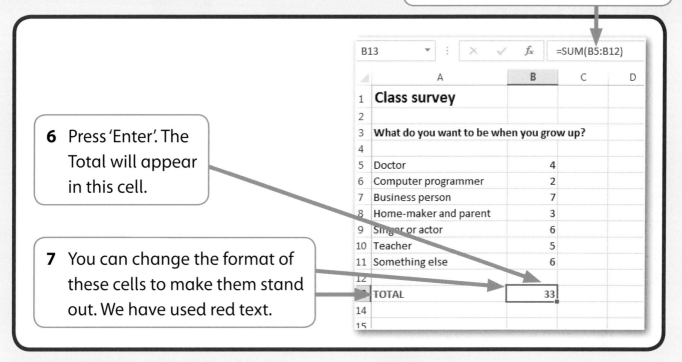

6 Press 'Enter'. The Total will appear in this cell.

7 You can change the format of these cells to make them stand out. We have used red text.

Activity   Calculate the total

1 Use the Sum function to calculate the total value for your spreadsheet.

2 Print the spreadsheet.

3 Remember to save your work.

 If you have time...

The AutoSum button lets you add other functions to your spreadsheet. These include average and maximum values.

Try out the different functions. See what results you get.

Click on this little arrow to open the list of functions.

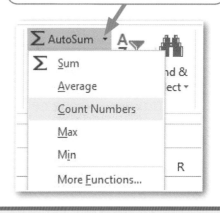

Talk about...

If you change the values in a spreadsheet, the results will change too.

You can test this. Change the values in your spreadsheet and the total value changes automatically.

Why is this useful in real life?

You will learn:

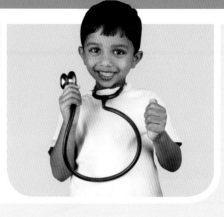

→ what a percentage is

→ what a spreadsheet formula is

→ how to make a spreadsheet formula

→ how to use a cell reference in a formula.

In this lesson you will use a spreadsheet **formula** to work out what **percentage** of students want to be a doctor.

> Half of 100 is 50, so 50% means 'one half'.

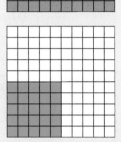

Percentages

A percentage is another way of showing a fraction. A percentage shows a fraction as an amount out of 100.

You can work out what percentage of a total any value is. You divide the value by the total.

> One quarter of 100 is 25, so 25% means 'one quarter'.

Spreadsheet formulas

A spreadsheet formula makes the computer carry out a calculation.

Every spreadsheet formula begins with an equals sign: ═══

Cell references

This is how to work out the percentage of students who want to be a doctor:

→ Start with the number of students who want to be a doctor.

→ Divide by the total number of students in the class survey.

To put a value from a cell into a formula, you need to use the cell reference. To do this just click on the cell that holds the value.

How to start the formula

The formula goes in the cell next to the number value. That is cell C5.

> Type an equals sign here to start the formula.

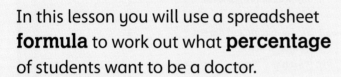

	A	B	C	D
1	**Class survey**			
2				
3	**What do you want to be when you grow up?**			
4				
5	Doctor		4	=
6	Computer programmer		2	
7	Business person		7	
8	Home-maker and parent		3	

How to put a cell reference in your formula

After the equals sign you will add a cell reference.

Cell B5 shows the number of students who want to be a doctor.

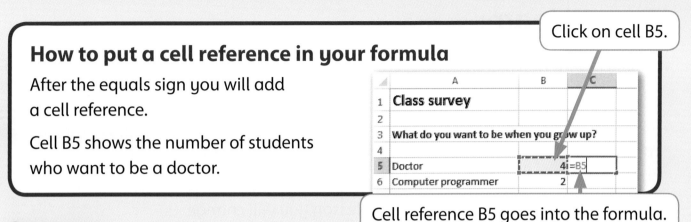

Click on cell B5.

Cell reference B5 goes into the formula.

Operators

Spreadsheet formulas include mathematical symbols. The most common mathematical symbols are:

+ add   − subtract   * multiply   / divide

In this formula you will use the division sign.

How to complete the formula

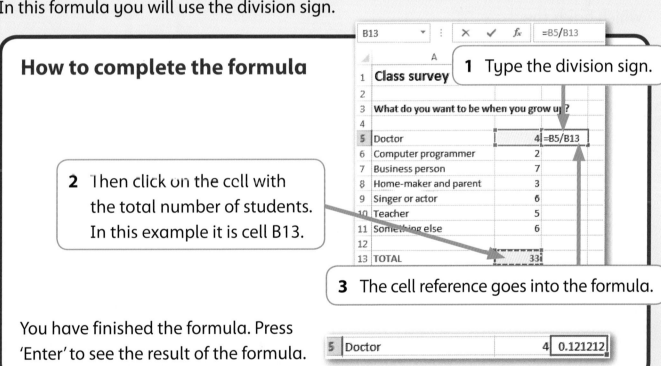

1 Type the division sign.

2 Then click on the cell with the total number of students. In this example it is cell B13.

3 The cell reference goes into the formula.

You have finished the formula. Press 'Enter' to see the result of the formula.

Activity   Make a spreadsheet formula

Use the instructions here to make the spreadsheet formula.

Remember to save your work.

You will learn:

→ how to format a value as a percentage.

> This result is a decimal.

In the last lesson you used a spreadsheet formula. You divided the number of students who want to be a doctor by the total number of students.

| 5 | Doctor | 4 | 0.121212 |

The result is shown as a decimal. In this lesson you will change this number into a percentage.

How to turn a decimal into a percentage

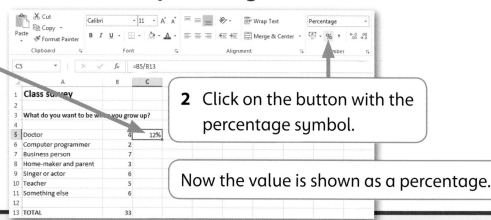

1 Select cell C5, which holds the decimal value.

2 Click on the button with the percentage symbol.

Now the value is shown as a percentage.

Activity | Practise your skills

You have learned how to make a formula to divide the number of students who want to be a doctor by the total number of students. You have learned how to format the result as a percentage.

1 Now practise your skills by entering a formula in the next cell down.

→ Put an equals sign in cell C6.

→ Click on cell B6.

→ Enter the division sign and then click on B13.

2 Then format this value as a percentage.

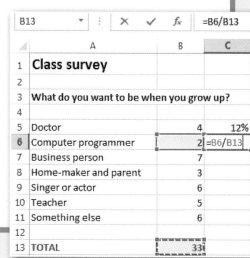

Activity | Enter more formulas

1 Enter a formula next to every number.

2 Format them all so that you see percentages.

3 Save and print your work.

	A	B	C
1	**Class survey**		
2			
3	**What do you want to be when you grow up?**		
4			
5	Doctor	4	12%
6	Computer programmer	2	6%
7	Business person	7	21%
8	Home-maker and parent	3	9%
9	Singer or actor	6	18%
10	Teacher	5	15%
11	Something else	6	18%
12			
13	TOTAL	33	

Talk about...

Percentages and fractions

Your teacher will give you a worksheet. It shows pie charts of different percentages. The blue sections show the percentages.

Remember that a percentage is a different way of writing a fraction.

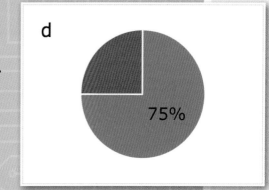

d

75%

Match the percentages to these fractions:

→ one half   → one third   → one fifth

→ one quarter   → three quarters   → one eighth.

You can work as a class or in a group.

If you have time...

1 Make changes to the numbers stored in the spreadsheet. You will see that all the percentages change automatically. Explore the effect of making changes.

2 a Sketch the pie charts on the worksheet. See how accurate you can be.

   b Draw a new pie chart to show the percentage that is the same as one tenth.

You will learn:

→ how we can use a pie chart to show data
→ how to make a pie chart.

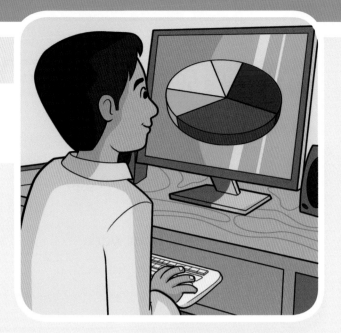

How pie charts show data

A slice of a pie chart stands for a fraction. The bigger the fraction, the bigger the slice. For example, the slice for one third is bigger than the slice for one quarter.

A **pie chart** is split into many slices to show how a total is made up of different values. Each slice of a pie chart is called a **segment**.

Now you will make a pie chart that shows the data in your spreadsheet.

How to select the data

First you must select the data for your chart. You must select:

→ the labels that show the different jobs

→ the numbers that show how many students chose each job.

Do not select the percentages. Do not select the total.

To select the data drag the cursor across all the cells.

	A	B	C
1	**Class survey**		
2			
3	**What do you want to be when you grow up?**		
4			
5	Doctor	4	12%
6	Computer programmer	2	6%
7	Business person	7	21%
8	Home-maker and parent	3	9%
9	Singer or actor	6	18%
10	Teacher	5	15%
11	Something else	6	18%
12			
13	TOTAL	33	
14			

Make sure all the cells you need are highlighted.

How to make a pie chart

The tools you need to make a pie chart from this data are on the 'Insert' tab at the top of the screen.

1 Click on the 'Insert' tab.

2 There are many different types of chart.

3 Click here to see the pie chart options.

4 We have chosen the chart called '3-D Pie'.

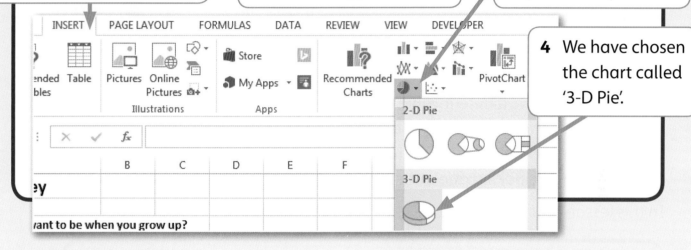

Activity Make a pie chart

Follow the instructions above to make a pie chart from your spreadsheet data.

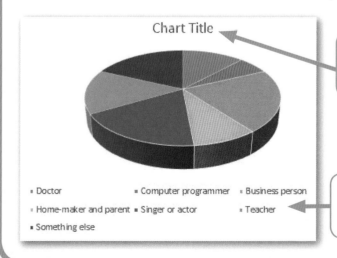

This is the 'Chart Title'. Select it and type a new title for the chart.

This is the key (or legend). It tells you what the different colours mean.

If you have time...

Try different designs for the pie chart. Which do you like best?

You will learn:

➔ how we can use a bar chart to show data
➔ how to make a bar chart.

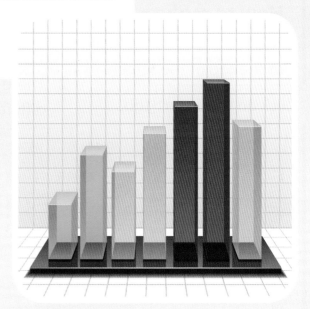

Bar charts

A **bar chart** is another way of comparing values. In the spreadsheet software a bar chart is called a column chart.

The bar chart shows different values using bars of different heights. We can use a bar chart to compare different values quickly by eye instead of looking at numbers.

In this lesson you will turn your pie chart into a bar chart.

How to change the chart type

1 Click on the chart to select it.

2 Open the 'Design' tab.

3 Click on 'Change Chart Type'.

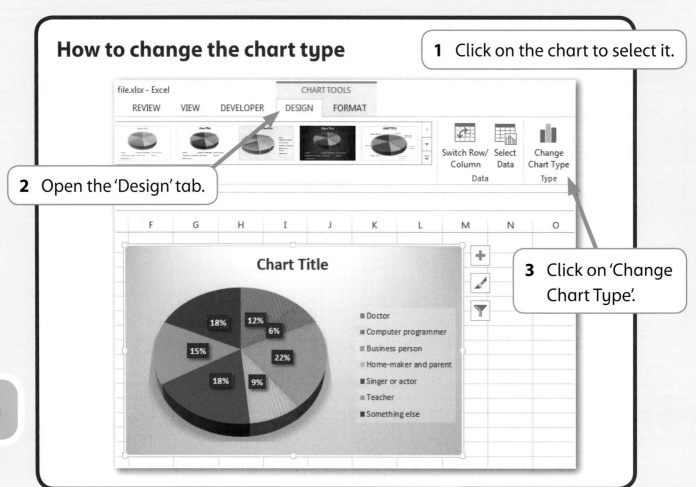

How to choose a bar chart

When you click on 'Change Chart Type' a new window opens. Choose the type of bar chart that you like.

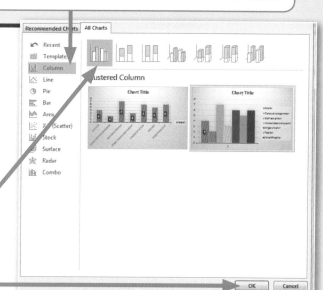

2 We have chosen this style.

3 Click 'OK' to finish.

How to pick a colour scheme

The 'Design' tab also lets you choose a colour scheme.

Click here to open a selection of colour schemes.

We have chosen these colours for this chart.

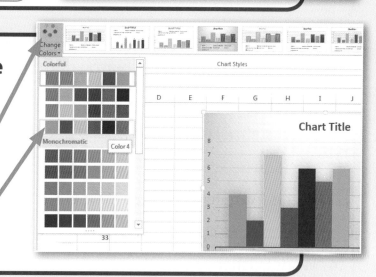

Activity **Make a bar chart**

1 Change your pie chart to a bar chart.

2 Choose the type of bar chart you like best. Choose a colour scheme for your bar chart.

3 Save and print your work to show what you have learned in this unit.

If you have time...

1 Try out different chart designs and colour schemes.

2 Change the values in the spreadsheet and see how the bar chart changes too.

3 Print every example that you make.

What you have learned about handling data

In this unit you have learned:

→ how to store number values using a spreadsheet

→ how to use spreadsheet functions

→ how to create spreadsheet formulas using cell references

→ how to make pie charts and bar charts that show your number values.

The activities on this page will let you see how much you have learned.

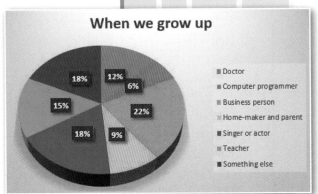

When we grow up

- Doctor
- Computer programmer
- Business person
- Home-maker and parent
- Singer or actor
- Teacher
- Something else

---

1 What does the AutoSum button do?   Σ AutoSum ▾

_____

2 What symbol comes at the start of every spreadsheet formula?

_____

3 In this formula what does 'E6' mean?   =E6/F6

_____

4 What fraction means the same as 33%?

_____

5 Explain how a chart helps you to understand and compare number values.

_____

_____

_____

6 Explain the difference between a pie chart and a bar chart.

_____

_____

_____

50

Activity Drinks for sports day

A teacher wants to give students drinks at the school sports day. She asks them what drink they like best. This spreadsheet shows their answers.

	A	B	C	D
1	Drinks for sports day			
2				
3	Cola	6		
4	Orange juice	7		
5	Water	3		
6	Strawberry milk	8		
7	Iced tea	5		

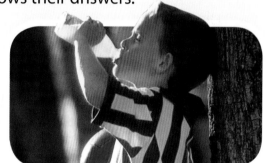

1 Make this spreadsheet.

2 Use a function to add up the total number of students.

3 Use formulas to work out the percentage of students who chose each drink.

4 If you have time, make a chart to show the data.

Activity Label the spreadsheet

Print out the spreadsheet you made in the practical activity. If you have not completed the activity, your teacher will give you this picture of a spreadsheet.

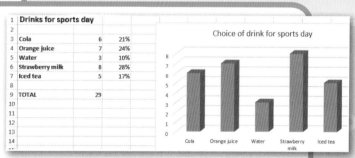

Follow these instructions and write a label for each thing.

1 Draw a circle round the data that was used to make the chart.

2 Draw an arrow to the cell that shows the result of the Sum function.

3 Draw an arrow to a cell that shows the result of a formula.

4 Draw an arrow to the bar in the bar chart that shows how many students chose orange juice.

51

4 Control the computer: Making a maths quiz

By the end of this unit you will:

→ know how to make and run a *Scratch* script for a quiz program

→ understand what input and output are

→ know how to make a program that reads input and makes output

→ know how to make the quiz program mark quiz answers as right or wrong

→ know how to make the quiz program keep score.

In this unit you are going to make a maths quiz using the computer language called *Scratch*.

Computer programs control the way that a computer operates. Different programs make the computer do different things. In this unit you will create a computer quiz game. The computer will ask questions, and say if the answer is right or wrong. It will show the score on the screen.

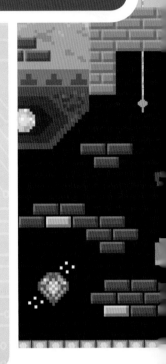

data
event   IF statement
input   output
logical test   run
sprite   script
variable   stage

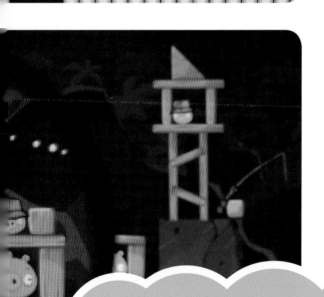

Talk about...

Sometimes your teacher sets a test in class.

1 What is the best thing about having a test? What is the worst thing?

2 Why do you think your teacher sets tests for the class?

3 If you were the teacher, would you stop having tests?

Activity | Maths questions

Before you begin, decide what maths questions you want to put into the quiz.

1 Write ten simple maths questions for younger children. Make a note of the right answer to each question.

2 Think of the hardest maths topic you have learned this year. Make a quiz with ten questions about that maths topic. Remember to note the right answers.

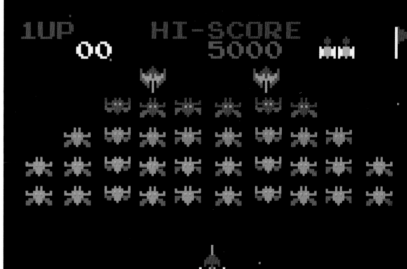

Fascinating fact

The first computer games were made in the 1950s, more than 60 years ago. The first game was noughts and crosses. There was also a tennis game and a spaceship game called 'Spacewar'. Not many people had computers in those days.

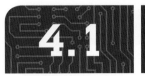

4.1 | A simple script

You will learn:

→ what *Scratch* is
→ what a script is
→ how to make and run a *Scratch* script.

Scratch is a programming language for young learners. In this unit you will learn to create simple programs using the *Scratch* programming language. You will create a simple maths quiz for younger students.

How to make a script in *Scratch*

A *Scratch* **script** is made of blocks. You make a script by fitting blocks together.

You always begin a script by choosing an **event**. An event is something that happens. When the event happens, the script will be carried out.

The blocks are different colours. 'Event' blocks are brown.

This is the script you will make. The script will be carried out when the **sprite** is clicked. The script tells the computer what to do.

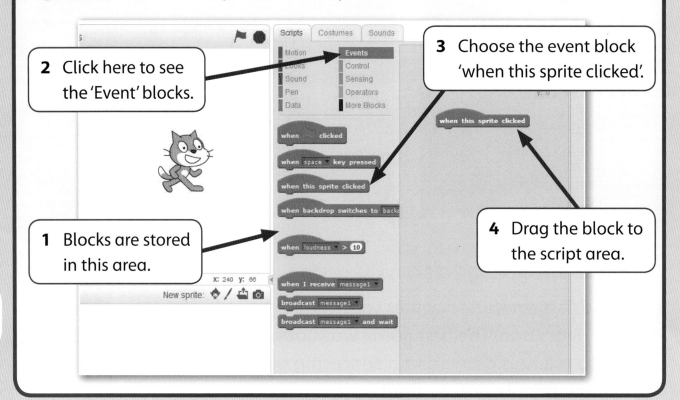

2 Click here to see the 'Event' blocks.

3 Choose the event block 'when this sprite clicked'.

1 Blocks are stored in this area.

4 Drag the block to the script area.

How to make the sprite ask you your name

Next, you will make the sprite 'talk' to you. It will ask what your name is and wait for an answer.

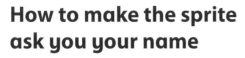

2 Pick this block.

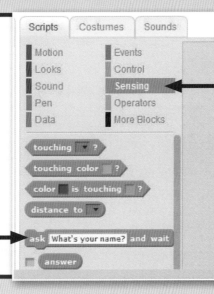

1 Click here to see the 'Sensing' blocks. They are light blue.

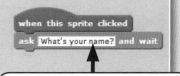

3 Drag it to the script area and join it to the 'Event' block.

How to run your script

You have made a simple *Scratch* script. Now you can **run** the script. This means the computer will carry out the script. You will see the sprite do the action.

1 Click here to make the **stage** bigger.

2 Click on the sprite to run the script.

3 Type your name and press 'Enter'.

When you run the script the sprite asks 'What's your name?'

Activity | Create a *Scratch* program

1 Create a *Scratch* program with these features:

→ There is a sprite.

→ When you click on the sprite it asks you your name.

2 Run the script to make sure it works.

3 Save your work.

You will learn:

→ what input and output are
→ how to make a program that reads input
  and makes output.

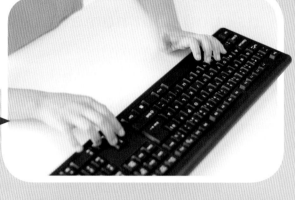

Input means any signal that goes IN to the computer. For example, typing into the computer or clicking on the sprite.

Output means anything that comes OUT of the computer. For example, a display on the screen, or a sound.

After this lesson your program will:

→ let you input your name

→ make the computer output your name.

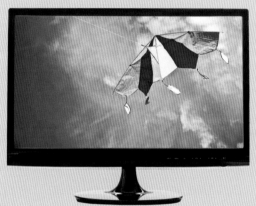

Open your script from the last lesson. When you run the program the sprite asks you for your name. You type your name and press 'Enter'. Your name is the input.

How to make the sprite say 'Hello!'

Now you will change the program so that the sprite says 'Hello!' The block you need is in the 'Looks' area. These blocks are purple.

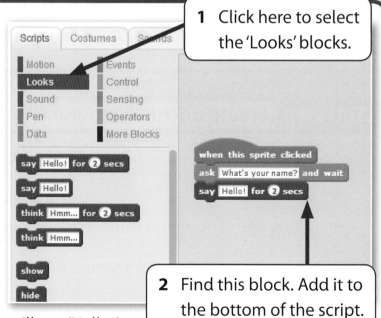

1 Click here to select the 'Looks' blocks.

2 Find this block. Add it to the bottom of the script.

Run the program now. The sprite will say 'Hello!'

How to make the sprite say your name

You can change the script so that the sprite says your name instead of 'Hello!'

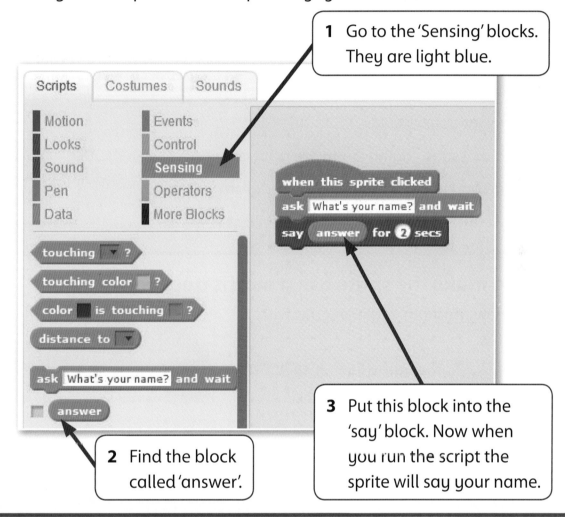

1 Go to the 'Sensing' blocks. They are light blue.

2 Find the block called 'answer'.

3 Put this block into the 'say' block. Now when you run the script the sprite will say your name.

Activity Make the sprite talk to you

1 Open the file you saved last time.

2 Add blocks to the script so the sprite says 'Hello!', then change the script so that the sprite says your name.

3 Try typing in different answers to the question. Whatever answer you type, the sprite will say that answer.

4 Save your work.

You will learn:

➔ what an IF statement is

➔ how to use IF to control output.

In the next two lessons you will make a new program. This program will:

➔ ask a simple maths question

➔ let you input your answer

➔ output a message saying if you are right or wrong.

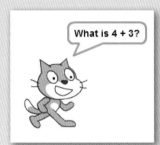

In this lesson you will start to build the program.

We will make the sprite ask the question **'What is 4 + 3?'**

How to make the sprite ask a maths question

Start a new program. Make a script with two blocks:

➔ the block 'when this sprite clicked'. It is in the brown 'Events' blocks.

➔ the block that asks a question. It is in the light blue 'Sensing' blocks.

Fit these two blocks together.

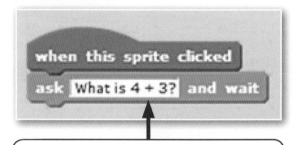

Delete the question 'What is your name?' Type 'What is 4 + 3?'

You want the computer to choose a reply.

➔ If you input the right answer, 7, the computer will say 'You are right'.

➔ If you input a different number, the computer will say 'You are wrong'.

An **IF statement** is a way to choose between two outputs. It has a test and two different outputs. The computer uses the test to choose which output to show.

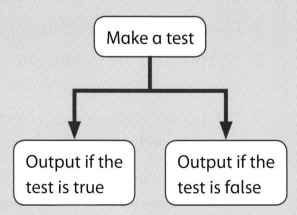

In this lesson you will put the two messages into the program.

In the next lesson you will make the test that chooses between the messages.

How to add an IF statement to your script

The 'IF' block is a 'Control' block. These blocks are yellow.

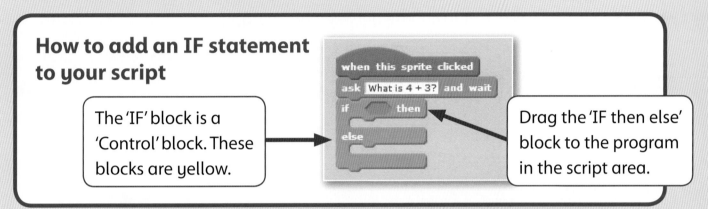

Drag the 'IF then else' block to the program in the script area.

The 'IF' block has two gaps in it. These gaps will hold the two different messages.

How to add messages to the IF statement

Find the purple 'Looks' block 'say Hello! for 2 seconds'. This makes the sprite say a message.

1 Drag one block here. Change the words to 'You are right'.

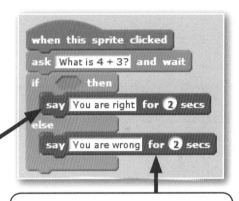

2 Drag another block here. Change the words to 'You are wrong'.

Activity | Add the IF statement

1 Create the program shown in this lesson. You can pick any simple maths question that you like.

2 Do not run the program yet. It will not work. You will finish the program in the next lesson.

3 Remember to save your work.

Talk about...

What messages do you want the computer to use to say if the answer is right or wrong?

You will learn:

→ what a logical test is

→ how to use a logical test to choose between two outputs.

In the last lesson you made a program that asked the question 'What is 4 + 3?'

We want the computer to check the user's answer to see if it is right or wrong. That is the test.

In this lesson you will add the test to the 'IF' block. That will make the quiz program work.

A computer is logical. The computer will use a **logical test**. This is a test with a simple Yes/No answer.

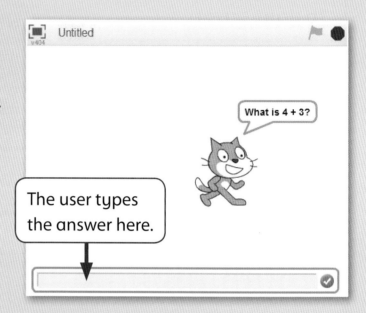

What is 4 + 3?

The user types the answer here.

How to add an operator that compares two values

You will use a green 'Operators' block. They let you join or compare two values.

Find the block with an equals sign in it. Drag it into the program.

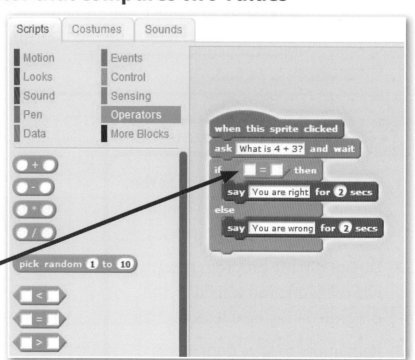

How to create the logical test

You have added an operator that compares two values. To create the logical test you must add the two values.

→ The first value is the user answer.

→ The second value is the number 7.

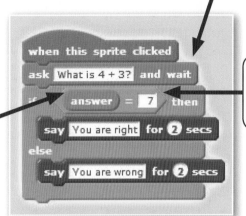

2 Drag the 'answer' block into the green 'Operator' block.

1 Look at the blue 'Sensing' blocks.

3 Enter the value 7.

Activity Create the logical test

1 Add the blocks shown on this page to make the complete program.

2 Save your completed program.

3 Run the program by clicking on the sprite.

4 Enter the right answer. What happens?

5 Enter the wrong answer. What happens?

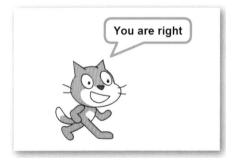

If you have time...

1 You can change the question that the sprite asks. Try this.

→ Change the question to 'What is 5 + 7?'

→ Change the right answer to 12.

2 Save the program with these changes. Click on the sprite to run the program.

3 Make the sprite ask different questions. Remember to change the logical test.

You will learn:

→ how to add new sprites to your program
→ how to copy a script to a new sprite.

 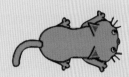 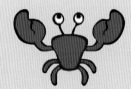 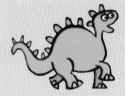

Now you will add lots of sprites to your program. Each sprite will ask a different maths question.

Here is some good news. You don't have to make the script again. You can copy the script to all the new sprites. All you need to change is the question each sprite asks.

How to add new sprites to your program

You can easily add new sprites to the program.

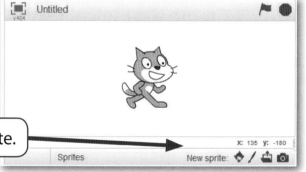

Click here to choose a new sprite.

You will see a library of sprites. A library is a collection of resources. Click on any sprite to add it to the program. We have chosen a butterfly.

Now the stage shows two sprites. You can drag them to any position.

The sprites are also shown below the stage. Pick a sprite by clicking on it. You will see the script for that sprite.

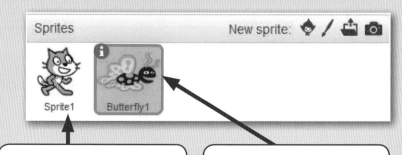

Click on the cat sprite. You will see the script for the cat sprite.

Click on the butterfly. It has no script.

How to copy your script to another sprite

You can copy the script from the cat to the butterfly.

Drag the script from the cat to the butterfly. Cover the butterfly with the script.

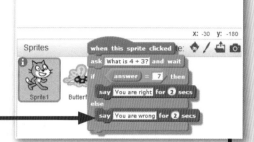

How to change the question

Now you can change the script so that the butterfly asks a different question.

1 Change the question in this block.

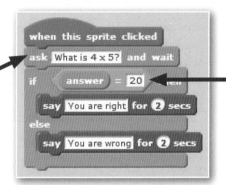

2 Change the right answer in the test block.

Activity **Add another sprite**

1 Add another sprite to the stage.

2 Copy the script onto the sprite.

3 Change the question and answer in the script.

4 Save the program.

5 Run the program. Click on the sprites and answer the questions.

Talk about...

Discuss the type of questions we can add to this program. Should they be hard or easy? Can we add questions that are not to do with maths?

If you have time...

Add lots of sprites to the program. Make each sprite ask a different question.

You will learn:

→ what a variable is

→ how to use a variable to store a changing value.

In this lesson you will make your program keep score. Every time you give the right answer your score will go up by one.

The score is an example of **data**. Data is the name for facts and figures. Data can be stored in the computer.

The score is stored as a **variable**. A variable is a value stored by the computer. As your score gets higher the value of the variable will change.

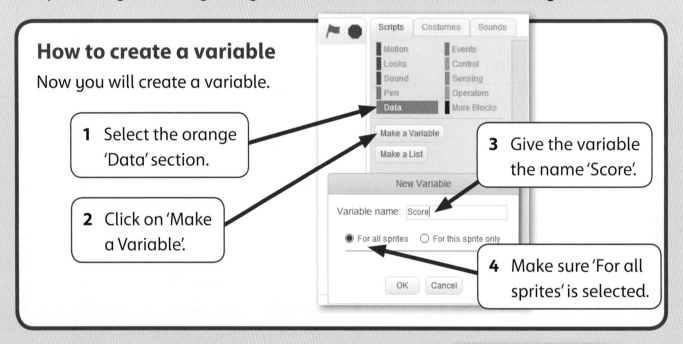

How to create a variable

Now you will create a variable.

1 Select the orange 'Data' section.

2 Click on 'Make a Variable'.

3 Give the variable the name 'Score'.

4 Make sure 'For all sprites' is selected.

Every variable must have a name. The name must tell you what the data is. You have made a variable called 'Score'.

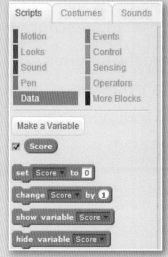

Some new blocks have appeared. You can use these blocks now.

How to make your program keep score

If the answer to a question is right, you want the score to go up by 1.

Find the block that says 'change Score by 1'. Now add that block to the script for one of your sprites.

Put the block into the 'IF' block in your script.

Make this change for every sprite.

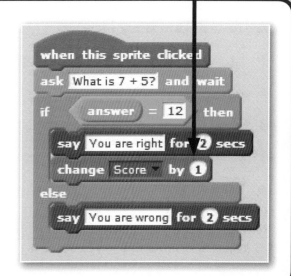

How to set the score to zero

When the quiz starts the score must be 0 (zero).

Look at the brown 'Events' blocks. Choose the first event, 'when green flag clicked'. This event will start the quiz game.

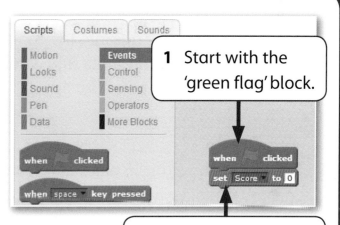

1 Start with the 'green flag' block.

2 Find this 'Data' block. It sets the score to 0.

Activity [Keep score]

1 Add commands to your program so that it keeps score.

2 Save your work.

3 Run the program. You can challenge your friends.

If you have time…

Make a large program with lots of different sprites.

What you have learned about making a maths quiz

In this unit you have learned:

→ how to make and run a *Scratch* script for a quiz program

→ what input and output are

→ how to make a program that reads input and makes output

→ how to make the quiz program mark quiz answers as right or wrong

→ how to make the quiz program keep score.

1 Every *Scratch* script starts with an event. Why does a script start with an event?

_____

_____

2 A student typed their age into the computer. The computer said 'Thank you'. What is the input and what is the output of this program?

_____

_____

3 The picture shows an 'IF' block. It has two spaces in it. Can you explain why the 'IF' block has two spaces?

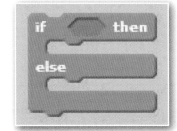

_____

_____

4 Why does an 'IF' block have a logical test in it?

_____

_____

5 A variable is used to store a value. How can you decide what name to give to the variable?

_____

_____

Activity | Label the picture

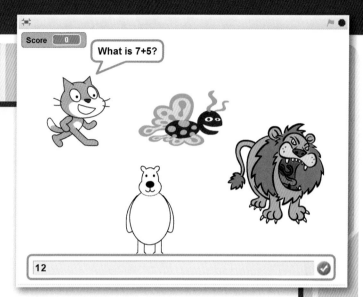

⬇ Your teacher will give you this picture.

1 Label these things in the picture:

- a sprite
- an example of user input
- an example of computer output.

2 Write the next message the sprite will say.

Activity | Change the quiz question

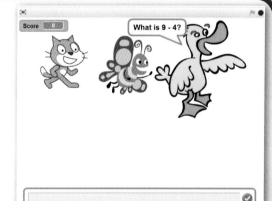

⬇ There is a file called *Sample Scratch quiz*. This is a maths quiz with some extra features.

1 Open this quiz game and play it by clicking on the sprites.

2 Make a note of what happens.

3 Edit the script of the cat sprite to change the question that it asks. Remember to change the IF test as well.

⏱ If you have time...

Add more sprites to the *Sample Scratch quiz*. Copy the script from the cat sprite to the new sprites you have added. Change the questions that they ask.

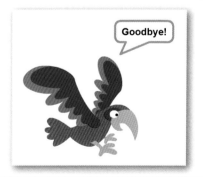

5 The Internet: Webquest!

By the end of this unit you will know:

→ how to do good searches online

→ how to spot sponsored links

→ how to search inside a website

→ how to check whether what a web page says is true

→ what makes a website helpful

→ how to reference the things you find online.

In this unit you are going to go on a webquest.

A quest is an adventurous journey where you search for something. In a **webquest**, you search for something on the internet.

Your webquest is to search for delicious dishes from around the world. You will use these to create a wonderful banquet menu for a great feast.

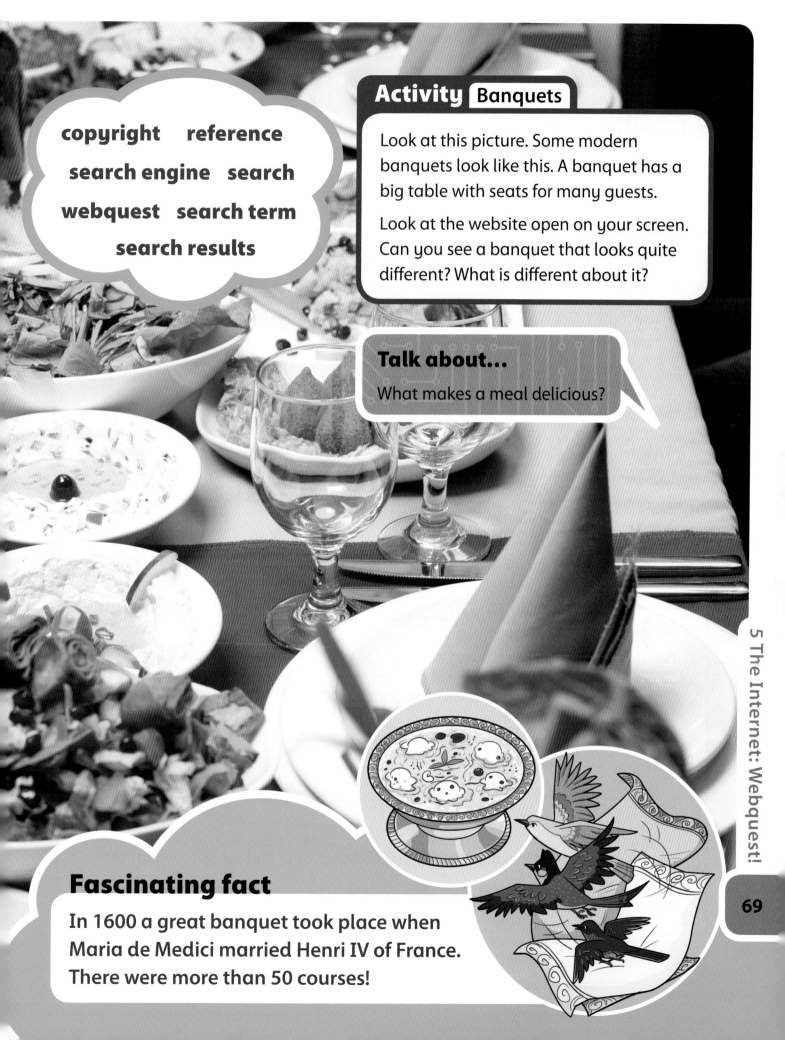

copyright   reference
search engine   search
webquest   search term
search results

Activity Banquets

Look at this picture. Some modern banquets look like this. A banquet has a big table with seats for many guests.

Look at the website open on your screen. Can you see a banquet that looks quite different? What is different about it?

Talk about...

What makes a meal delicious?

Fascinating fact

In 1600 a great banquet took place when Maria de Medici married Henri IV of France. There were more than 50 courses!

You will learn:

→ how to do good searches online.

Every time we **search** for something online there are thousands of web pages we could look at.

We need to have clever ways of making our searches clearer, so that we find the information we want.

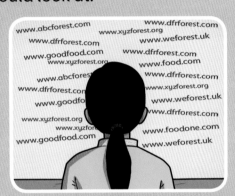

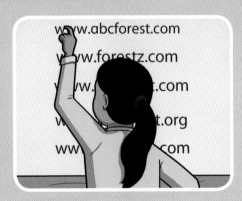

How to use clear search terms

To find what you are looking for on the internet, you need to make sure your **search terms** are very clear.

Use the right number of words.

Choose the words for your search term carefully.

Use " " around your search term. These are called quotation marks.

Try this.

1 Type this search term into your **search engine**.

> dessert 🔍

Press 'Enter'.

Look at the first three **search results**. Are they useful for your webquest?

2 Now type this search term.

> dessert recipe Argentina 🔍

Press 'Enter'.

We do not need to type 'from'.

Are these results useful for your webquest?

3 Now type this search term and use quotation marks.

"Argentinian desserts"	🔍

The search engine will search for this exact phrase.

Press 'Enter'.

Are these results useful for your webquest?

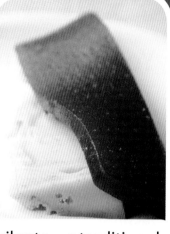

▲ Vigilante – a traditional Argentinian dessert

Activity   Delicious dishes

⬇ Work in your group. Look at the tasks on the *Information sheet*.

→ Find two different recipes for the same dish. Write a short report on which recipe you will choose and why.

→ Watch two online cooking videos. Compare them. Write a short report on which one you think is more interesting and useful, and why.

→ Write an information sheet about your dish for the banquet guests.

1 In your group, choose a type of recipe to search for. Try using the right number of words, the correct words and quotation marks.

You could use a web tool such as *Delicious* to bookmark sites you find useful.

2 Make a list of the search terms you use.

3 Choose the dish your group will provide for the banquet menu.

🕐 If you have time...

We can also use synonyms to help us. Try using a synonym for your search term. For example, if your word is 'dessert', try 'pudding'.

A synonym is a word that means the same as another word.

Talk about...

Share your most useful search term with the rest of your class. Why was it most useful?

You will learn:

→ how to do good searches online
→ how to spot sponsored links.

You already know three ways of making your searches better. Can you remember them?

Here are two more tips.

| Beware of sponsored links. | → ⬚ ← | Use a minus sign. |

Sponsored links

⬇ Some companies pay the search engine to have sponsored links or sponsored advertisements. This means that links to these companies' websites will appear at the top of the page of search results.

They might still be useful, but they might be trying to sell you something you don't need. So be careful.

How to use the minus sign in your search terms

Use the minus sign before a word to show that you don't want the search engine to look for that word. For example, if you don't like cheese you can search for recipes with no cheese in them.

1 Type this search term.

Press 'Enter'.

What links do you see?

> salad recipe ⚲

> **Salad Recipes** - Allrecipes.com
> Find the best green **salad recipes**, plus trusted recipes for more than 3220 other dinner and picnic salads.
> allrecipes.com/recipes/salad/
>
> Quick & Delicious Summer **Salad Recipes** - Southern Living
> Fresh, easy, and pretty enough for a party – these colorful chicken **salad recipes**, potato **salad recipes**, berry **salad recipes**, shrimp **salad recipes** and coleslaw ...
> www.southernliving.com/food/entertaining/cool-summer-salads
>
> Green **Salad Recipes** - Allrecipes.com
> The best **salads** for bagged mixed greens or whole heads. **Recipes** for spinach **salad**, Greek **salad**, and more.
> allrecipes.com/recipes/salad/green-salads/

2 Now type this search term.

Press 'Enter'.

What links do you see?

| salad recipe -cheese | 🔍 |

Homestyle Potato Salad
Apr 4, 2014 ... This Homestyle Potato **Salad** is my Mom's **recipe**. I've never had potato **salad** that comes CLOSE to being as good as hers, she just knows how ...
www.favfamily**recipes**.com/homestyle-potato-**salad**.html

Tofu Avocado Salad Recipe | Fresh Tastes Blog | PBS Food
Aug 21, 2012 ... When a regular **salad** leaves you unsatisfied, try this tofu avocado **salad recipe** instead for a filling lunch. Get the **recipe** at PBS Food.
www.pbs.org/food/fresh-tastes/tofu-avocado-**salad**/

Healthy Salad Recipes - Cooking Light
Starters, sides, and easy weeknight dinners: Savor a seriously tasty **salad** with all the flavors you love and the convenience you need.
www.cookinglight.com/food/**recipe**-finder/healthy-**salad**-**recipes**

Cucumber Salad Recipes
Results 1 - 10 of 334 ... Try new ways of preparing cucumbers with cucumber **salad recipes**

Activity [Use the minus sign]

 1 Work in your group on your webquest task.

2 Use the minus sign to help you with your online searches.

3 Save your work in the group shared folder.

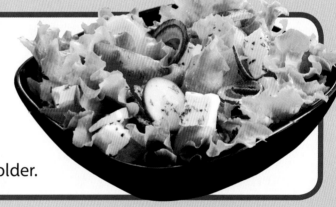

 If you have time...

1 You can use the plus sign to help you search too. The plus sign means that the search *must* have that word in it.

For example, searching for 'salad +tomato' means you will get web pages that have the word 'tomato' in them.

2 When you find some text or a picture online that you want to use in your work, make a note of where you found it. You will need this information later.

You will learn:

➔ how to search inside a website.

Sometimes we do not want to search the whole internet. We might just want to search inside a website that we know.

This chef is looking for a recipe that has rice in it.

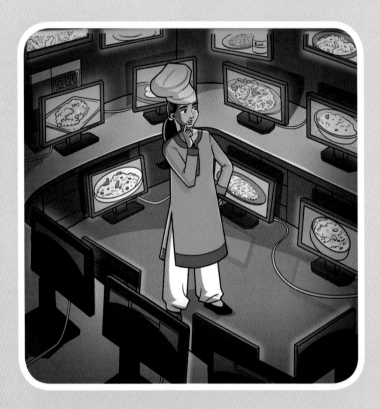

She could search the whole internet.

Or she could search one website that has lots of different recipes on it.

She decides that her recipe must be vegetarian. So she wants to search inside a vegetarian website.

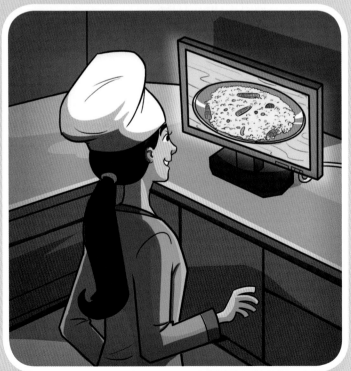

How to do a deep search of one website

1 Type 'site:' You do not need a space or a full stop.

3 Then type your search term.

site:vegetarianrecipe.com rice 🔍

2 Then type the URL of the website you'd like to search. You do not need to type 'www'.

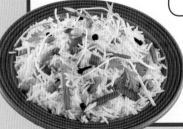 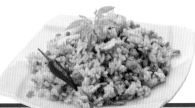

Activity Site search 1

1 Go to this website: www.food.com

2 Does this website have your group's recipe on it? Does it have recipes that use the same ingredients?

Do a deep site search to find out.

Activity Site search 2

1 Now carry on with your webquest projects in your group.

2 Use deep site searches to help you with your research.

3 Save your work in the group shared folder.

 If you have time...

What happens if you use quotation marks around a search term in a site search?

You will learn:

➜ how to check whether facts on a website are true.

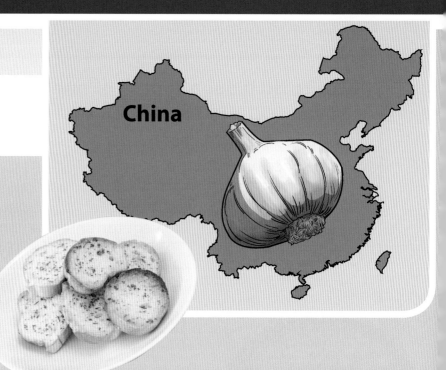

China

This is a fact:

> Most of the world's garlic comes from China.

This is an opinion:

> Most food tastes nicer if it has garlic in it.

Some websites are mainly fact.
Some websites are mainly opinion.

Some websites make money by including adverts, like this one for Gavin's Garlic Bread.

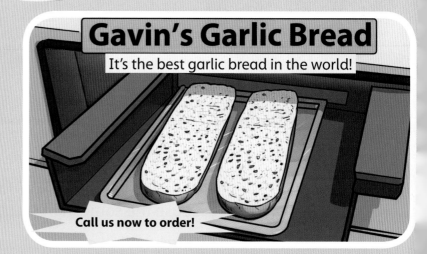

Gavin's Garlic Bread
It's the best garlic bread in the world!

Call us now to order!

How to check information we find online

Read the three statements about chopping onions at the top of page 77.

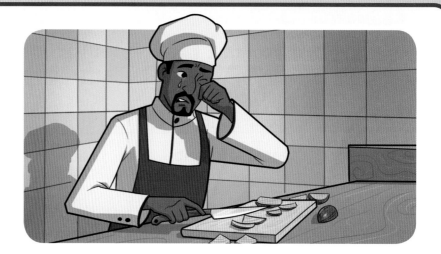

1 When we cut an onion, our eyes make tears because we feel sorry for the onion.

2 When we cut an onion, a gas escapes from the onion and gets into our eyes. Our eyes make tears to wash the gas away.

3 When we cut an onion, the onion sends small spikes into our eyes. Our eyes make tears because it is painful.

Ask yourself these checking questions:

➔ Has the information or website come from your teacher?

➔ Who has written and owns the website? Can you trust them?

➔ Can you check whether what the website says is true?

Which statement do you think is fact?

Look at these websites to check.

> When in doubt, check it out!

http://recipes.howstuffworks.com/question539.htm

http://www.scientificamerican.com/article/what-is-the-chemical-proc/

http://onions-usa.org/faqs/why-do-your-eyes-water-when-you-cut-onions

Talk about...

Which of the websites do you think you can trust the most?

Activity | Webquest continued

1 Now work in your group to continue your webquest.

2 Ask yourself the checking questions about each website you use.

3 Save your work in the group folder.

If you have time...

Look at the Wikipedia entry for 'banquet'. How much of this entry do you think is fact, and how much of it is opinion?

You will learn:

→ what makes a helpful website.

A helpful website is easy to use and well organised. It has the information that we want and the information is true.

A search engine cannot tell whether a website is helpful. Every time we browse the internet, we need to decide if a website will be helpful to us.

How to decide if a website is helpful

Ask yourself these questions about the website.

Can you find your way around the site? Can you easily find the information you are looking for?

Are there any sentences that you already know are true?

Are there any adverts?

Is the information on the site up to date?

What can you learn from the web address?

Can you contact the website owner?

Who is the writer? Can you trust them?

Does the website look organised?

Is there a good mix of pictures and words?

Who looks after the website? Can you trust them?

Activity Give it a score

1 Look at the main website you have used in your webquest.
Give it a score out of 5 for each of these questions:

→ Does the website look organised?

→ Is there a good mix of pictures and words?

→ Can you find your way around the site?

→ Is it free of adverts?

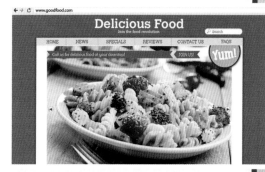

2 You should be reaching the end of your webquest now.

Use your time to finish your tasks.

3 Save your work in the group shared folder.

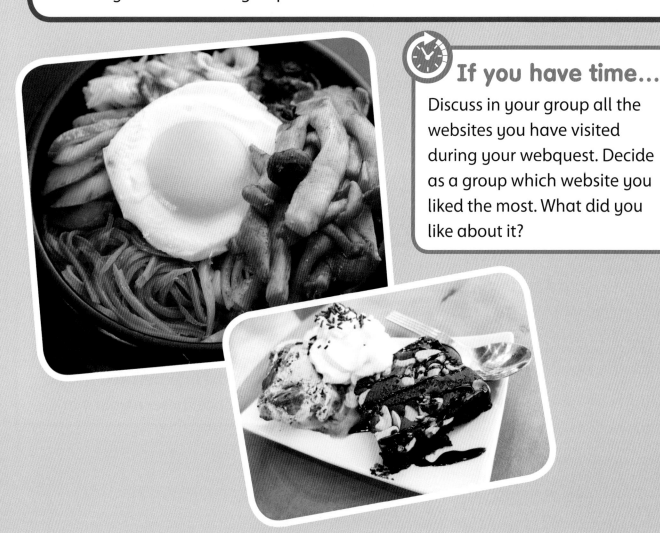

If you have time...

Discuss in your group all the websites you have visited during your webquest. Decide as a group which website you liked the most. What did you like about it?

You will learn:

→ how to reference the things you find online.

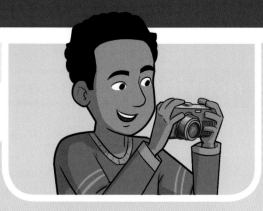

Mika used his new digital camera to take a photograph of his birthday celebration meal.

He was very proud of his photo. He decided to put it on his website.

Jay saw the photo and liked it too. He copied the photo and shared it on his website. Many people thought that Jay had taken the photo. This made Mika feel sad.

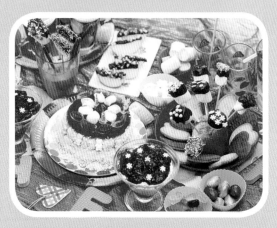

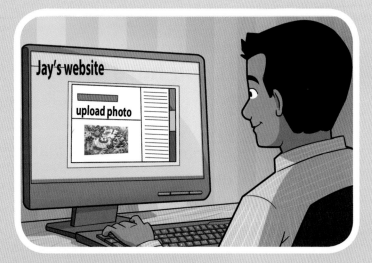

Jay's website

upload photo

When we create something, we usually own it. This is called **copyright**.
It means other people:

→ cannot copy our work

→ must ask our permission if they want to share our work

→ must say who created the work

→ cannot make any money from using our work.

Talk about...

Why was Mika sad?

What could he have done differently?

What could Jay have done differently?

If you have time...

Did you use any text or images from the internet? You should reference these in your work.

This is the copyright symbol.

After the copyright symbol you write the name of the person who made the work, and the date.

Look at page 82 of this book. Can you find the copyright symbol?

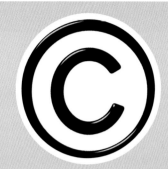

How to reference someone's work

Sometimes we want to use another person's work, for example a drawing, a photo, a poem or a story. When we do this, we need to **reference** the work. This means we need to say where we found it.

You can reference by:

→ writing the web address where you found the work

→ writing the name of the person who made the work you have used.

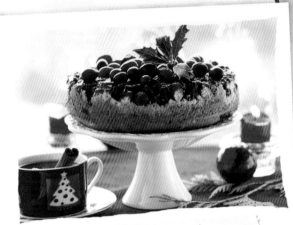

From: www.deliciousfoodrecipes.com

Activity | Webquest success!

1 Finish your last webquest tasks.

2 Add a copyright symbol to the bottom of your written work. Type (c). It automatically changes to a © symbol. Write your name after the symbol to show that this is your work.

3 Save your work in the group shared folder.

4 Share what you have done with the rest of the class.

5 Agree what the final banquet menu will be.

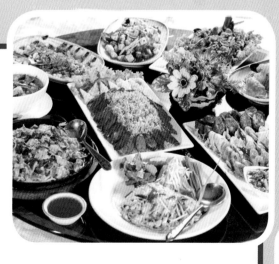

What you have learned about the internet

In this unit you have learned:

→ how to do good searches online

→ how to spot sponsored links

→ how to search inside a website

→ how to check whether facts on a website are true

→ what makes a website helpful

→ how to reference the things you find online.

1 Five of these sentences are ways of making your online search better. Write them down.

Choose the words for your search term carefully.

Use a minus sign.

Use quotation marks.

Use as many search terms as you can think of.

Use the right number of words.

Click on the most popular link.

Click on the first link that you see.

Be careful of sponsored links.

Put a question mark at the end of your search terms.

_____

_____

_____

_____

_____

2 Which of these search terms is the correct way to search inside a website?

a | site:deliciousfood.com apples | 🔍

b | site:www.deliciousfood.com apples | 🔍

c | site:deliciousfood.com.apples | 🔍

d | site;deliciousfood.com apples | 🔍

Activity   Sharing on the internet

1 You have invented a wonderful new recipe for ice cream. You want to share your recipe on the internet, but you don't want other people to use your recipe without saying you created it.

Explain to your teacher how you can do this.

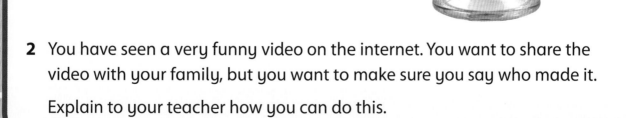

2 You have seen a very funny video on the internet. You want to share the video with your family, but you want to make sure you say who made it.

Explain to your teacher how you can do this.

6 Computers in society: A history of computing

By the end of this unit you will know:

→ about important inventions and ideas that have led to computers today

→ about seven important people in the history of computing

→ why it is important to be responsible when we use computers.

invention   algebra
binary   program
algorithm
responsible
internet
cipher/code

In this unit you are going to make a timeline for your classroom about the history of computing.

We are going to learn about the important people and inventions that have led to modern computers and the internet.

Talk about...

What do you think the Antikythera Mechanism is made of?

Do you think it looked like this when it was new?

Activity [Timeline]

Look at the image on this page. It shows the Antikythera Mechanism. It is a very ancient machine from about 70 BCE. We think it was used to predict when eclipses of the moon or sun would happen, but we don't really know.

→ Make a class timeline to show 70 BCE.

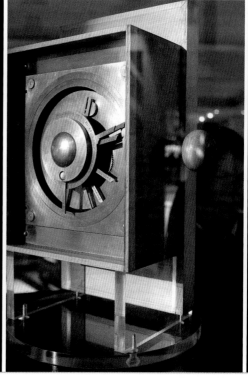

⚠ This is what we think the machine might have looked like.

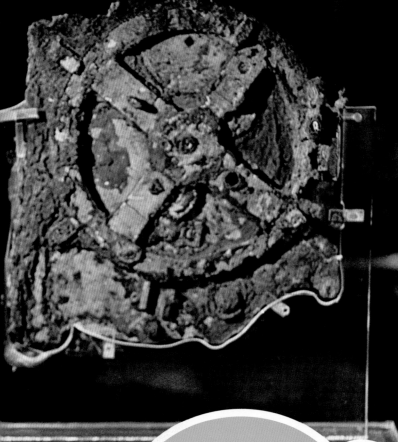

Fascinating fact

There were many people making interesting things at the same time as the Antikythera Mechanism was made. Important places were Corinth, Rhodes and Pergamum.

Pergamum

Corinth

Rhodes

Antikythera

You will learn:

➜ what an algorithm is

➜ why algorithms are important in computing

➜ about the person who invented the first algorithm.

Euclid lived such a long time ago that we don't know very much about his or her life.

Say Euclid like this: **You-klid.**

We don't even know whether Euclid was just one person or a group of people.

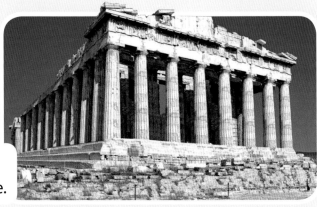

▶ We know that Euclid lived in about 300 BCE in ancient Greece.

Euclid wrote very important books about mathematics, and invented **algorithms**.

What is an algorithm?

An algorithm is a set of rules, steps or instructions.

We use algorithms in computing to tell computers what to do. They are very, very important.

A good algorithm describes each step in the instructions carefully and clearly.

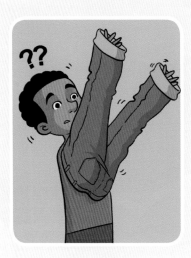

Put on underwear

↓

Put on trousers

↓

Put on top

↓

Put on socks

↓

Put on shoes

▲ If you miss out an instruction or get things in the wrong order the computer will get confused. Just like we do!

▲ This is a flowchart. It shows the order we put on our clothes. Computers use instructions in a special order too.

Activity 1 Follow the leader

Work with a partner. Your teacher will give one of you a picture.

Student 1:
Give instructions to your partner so they can draw the picture. You must not say what the object is.

Student 2:
Follow your partner's instructions to draw the picture.

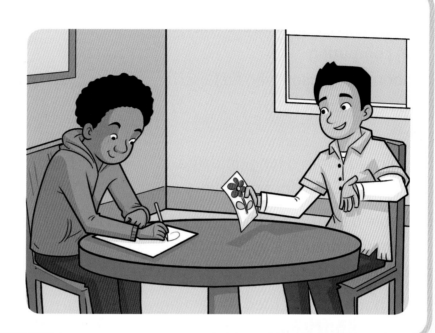

Activity 2 Euclid poster

Make a small poster about Euclid and algorithms for your class timeline. Your poster can have:

➜ the name 'Euclid' as the title

➜ one interesting fact about Euclid

➜ a picture of something from ancient Greece

➜ the word 'algorithm'.

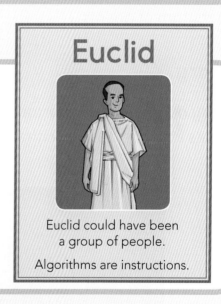

Euclid

Euclid could have been a group of people.

Algorithms are instructions.

If you have time...

Write a list of instructions for making a sandwich.

You have written an algorithm.

Talk about...

Do you think mathematics is important in computing?

You will learn:

→ what binary numbers are
→ why binary numbers are important in computing
→ about the person who first used binary numbers.

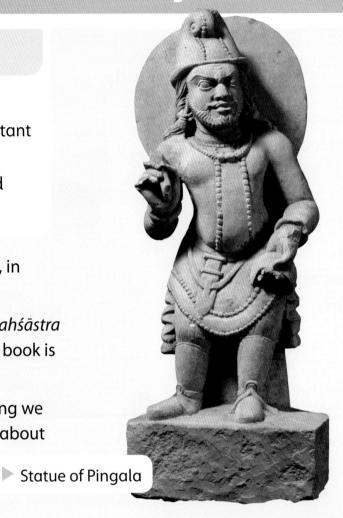

Pingala was born a long time ago, in about 200 BCE in ancient India.

He wrote a book called the *Chandahśāstra* in a language called Sanskrit. The book is about poetry.

In the book Pingala used something we now call **binary** numbers to talk about the rhythm of poems.

▶ Statue of Pingala

Binary

Binary numbers are important for computing because computers use electronic circuits that can only be either on or off.

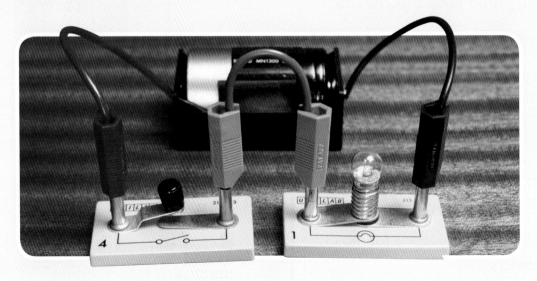

Binary numbers use 0 and 1 to represent all the numbers. When we use binary in computing, 'on' is a 1 and 'off' is a 0 (zero).

Activity | Signalling numbers

Work with a partner. Use a torch to signal numbers to each other.
Just like a computer, the torch is either off (for zero) or on (for 1).

→ How can you signal the number 5 to each other?

→ Think of two more numbers to signal to each other.

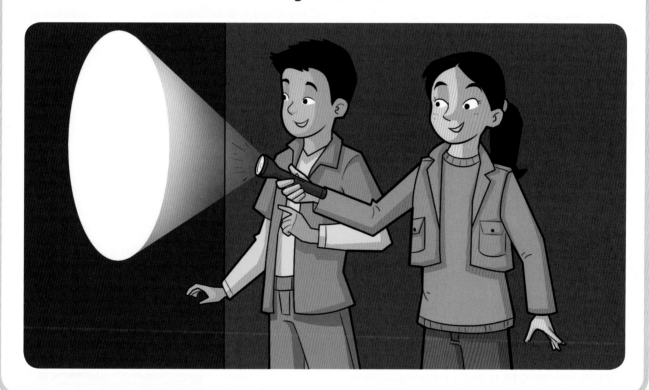

Activity | Pingala poster

Make a small poster about Pingala and binary numbers for your class timeline.

 If you have time...

How can you signal a large number, like 100 or 500?

Talk about...

Look at where Pingala is on your class timeline. Look at where Euclid is. Which of the two is older – Pingala or Euclid?

You will learn:

→ what algebra is
→ why algebra is important in computing
→ about the person who first used algebra to solve practical problems.

Al-Khwarizmi was a mathematician, astronomer and geographer. We think he came from ancient Arabia. He lived in about 800 CE.

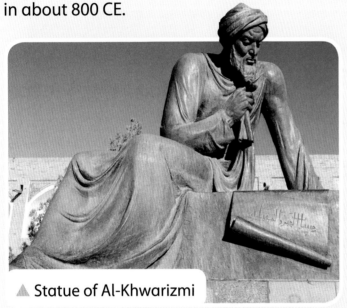

▲ Statue of Al-Khwarizmi

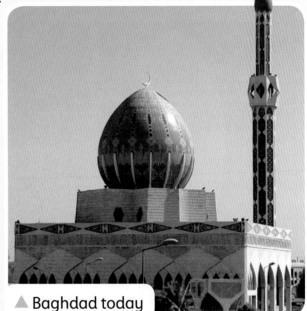

▲ Baghdad today

He worked in the House of Wisdom in Baghdad. He wrote a very famous book about mathematics. In this book he showed how to use mathematics to solve many different problems.

Al-Khwarizmi used **algebra** to solve these problems.

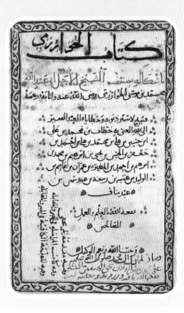

Activity Al-Khwarizmi poster

Make a small poster about al-Khwarizmi for your class timeline.

▲ A page from Al-Khwarizmi's book

Talk about...

What does 'wisdom' mean?

What do you think people did in the ancient House of Wisdom?

How to use algebra

Algebra is about solving problems with numbers, letters and symbols.

Using algebra to solve problems helps us do many things. It helps us make better internet search engines and make computers work faster.

In algebra we sometimes use symbols to mean numbers. Here is an example:

+ 3 = 10

So   = 7

Because 7 + 3 = 10

Activity Symbols

Write what each symbol is worth in each of these examples.

a 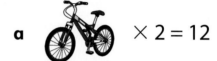 $\times 2 = 12$

=

b $+ 8 = 13$

=

c $+$ $= 8$

=

If you have time...

Can you create your own algebraic picture sum?

You will learn about:

→ Charles Babbage and the first computer

→ Ada Lovelace and the first computer program.

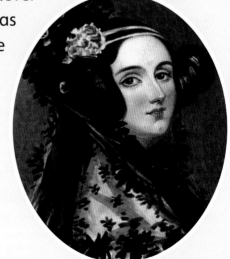

Charles Babbage (1791–1871) was a mathematician, philosopher, engineer and inventor from England.

His important **invention** was the Analytical Engine, which he designed in the 1830s. This was a machine that used cogs to work out complicated calculations. We now think of his machine as the first computer.

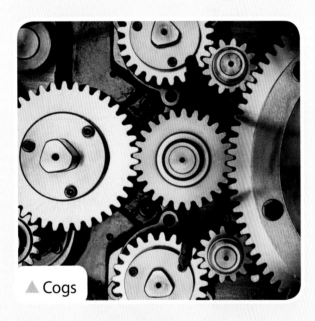

▲ Cogs

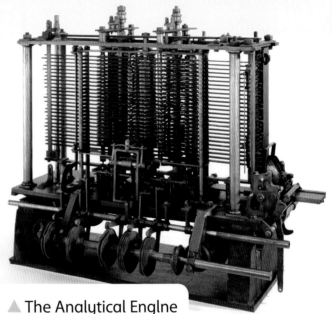

▲ The Analytical Engine

He worked with Ada Lovelace (1815–1852), who was a clever mathematician. She realised that Babbage's machine was not just useful for working with numbers, but could solve almost any problem.

Lovelace wrote some algorithms for the Analytical Engine. We now think of her algorithms as the first computer **programs**.

 Remember, an algorithm is a set of rules, steps or instructions.

How to use cogs to solve maths problems

Imagine a cog that can turn ten times. You can use the cog to do this sum:

$$3 + 4 =$$

The cog turns three times, and then another four times. So the answer to the sum is:

$$3 + 4 = 7$$

Talk about...

Ada Lovelace is the only female inventor in this book. Why do you think that is?

Activity Cogs

Work with a partner to make two cogs.

1 Cut out the cog shapes in the card your teacher has given you.

2 Make a hole in the middle of each cog.

3 Push a pencil through each hole.

4 Hold the cogs close to each other. Can you make them work?

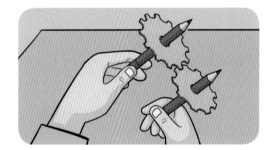

Activity Babbage and Lovelace poster

Make a small poster about Babbage and Lovelace for your class timeline.

If you have time...

Babbage used cards with holes in them to input numbers and instructions into his Analytical Engine.

Why do you think cards with holes in them work well with binary numbers?

93

You will learn:

→ about code-breaking and computing
→ what the Turing Test is
→ how to write and solve code messages.

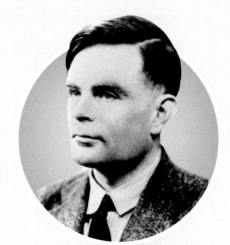

Alan Turing was a mathematician, computer scientist and philosopher. He lived in England between 1912 and 1954.

During World War II, Turing worked at the British code-breaking centre at Bletchley Park. The people there tried to decode the secret messages that were being sent about the war. These secret messages were called **ciphers** or **codes**.

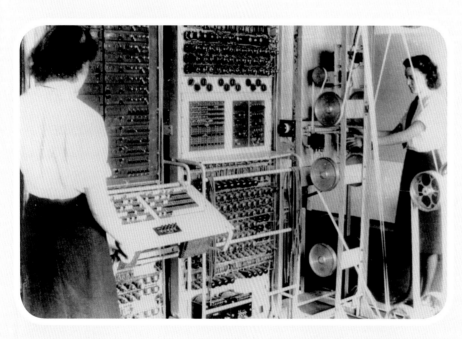

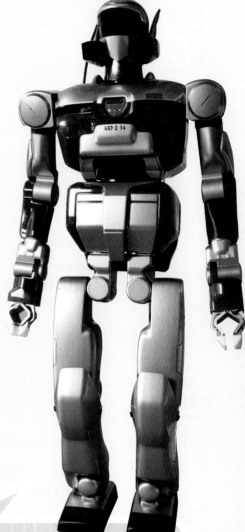

Turing invented the Turing Test in 1950. This test is not like an exam. It is a test that works out whether a computer can 'think' in the same way as a human can.

Talk about...

Do you think that one day we will have robots that think exactly like humans?

One of Turing's jobs during the war was to break some very difficult code messages called the Enigma codes.

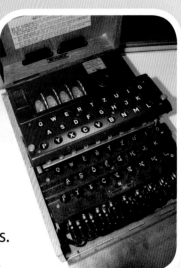

▶ This is the Enigma machine. It was used in World War II for making and breaking codes. Turing was able to break the Enigma codes.

How to be a code-breaker

Here is a message, hidden in a code.

SVOOL. GSRH RH Z XLWV.

In this code, the alphabet is reversed. A becomes Z, B becomes Y and so on.

A	B	C	D	E	F	G	H	I	J	K	L	M	N	O	P	Q	R	S	T	U	V	W	X	Y	Z
Z	Y	X	W	V	U	T	S	R	Q	P	O	N	M	L	K	J	I	H	G	F	E	D	C	B	A

So the code means: **Hello. This is a code.**

Activity Code-breaking

Write your own secret message using the reverse alphabet code. Give it to another person in the class to decode.

Activity Turing poster

Make a small poster about Turing for your class timeline.

If you have time...

⬇ Look at the worksheet *Code wheel* and make your own code wheel.

You will learn:

→ about the person who invented the internet

→ why we need to be responsible when we use computers and the internet.

Tim Berners-Lee was born in 1955 in Britain. He is a software engineer and a computer scientist.

In the 1980s Berners-Lee worked in CERN, an important laboratory in Switzerland.

He invented 'hypertext' to help scientists share information.

In 1989 he wrote a paper called 'Information Management: A Proposal'. He wrote about his idea for sharing information across the whole world. He called this the 'world wide web'.

The world's first website was launched in 1991. It was http://info.cern.ch. This was the start of the **internet**.

▲ The CERN laboratory

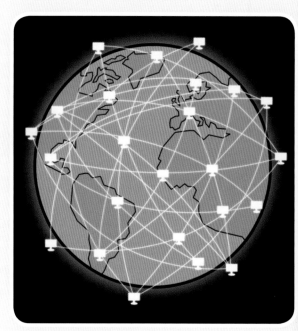

▲ The internet links computers all around the world.

```
                       WORLD WIDE WEB

The WorldWideWeb (W3) is a wide-area hypermedia[1] information retrieval
initiative aiming to give universal access to a large universe of documents.

Everything there is online about W3 is linked directly or indirectly to this
document, including an executive summary[2] of the project, Mailing lists[3] ,
Policy[4] , November's W3 news[5] , Frequently Asked Questions[6] .

     What's out there?[7]Pointers to the world's online information,
                   subjects[8] , W3 servers[9], etc.

     Help[10]          on the browser you are using

     Software         A list of W3 project components and their current
     Products[11]     state. (e.g. Line Mode[12] ,X11 Viola[13] ,
                      NeXTStep[14] , Servers[15] , Tools[16] , Mail
                      robot[17] , Library[18] )

     Technical[19]    Details of protocols, formats, program internals
                      etc

<ref.number>, <RETURN> for more, Quit, or Help:
```

▲ The very first web page

Talk about...

How did people find out information before the internet?

There are many people in the world who do not have internet access. What is life like for them?

Is the internet always a good thing?

How to use the internet responsibly

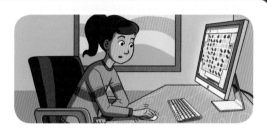

We need to be **responsible** when we use the internet. We need to be safe and to make good choices.

For example, this girl likes playing computer games on the internet.

Playing games with other people is fun.

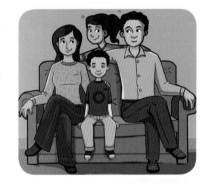
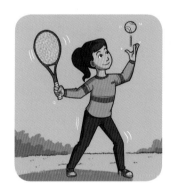

But she needs to make sure she doesn't spend so much time on her games that she forgets things like her family, hobbies and homework.

Activity   Tim Berners-Lee poster

Make a small poster about Tim Berners-Lee for your class timeline. Complete your other posters.

If you have time...

How many years are there between Euclid in 300 BCE and Tim Berners-Lee in 1991?

Can you imagine what computing will be like 2,000 years in the future?

What will have changed?

What you have learned about computers in society

In this unit you have learned:

→ about important inventions and ideas that have led to computers today

→ about important people in the history of computing

→ that we need to be thoughtful when we use computers

The activities on these pages will let you see how much you have learned.

---

1 Match the name of each person with the correct picture and with the correct invention.

1 Turing   **2** Al-Khwarizmi   **3** Babbage   **4** Lovelace   **5** Pingala

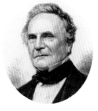 A

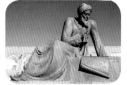 B

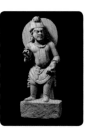 C

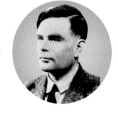 D

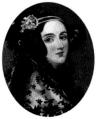 E

a First computer   **b** First computer program   **c** Algebra   **d** Binary numbers   **e** A test to see if a computer can 'think'

2 Copy the text and write the words in the right places.

Euclid   computers   internet   responsible   world   negative   thousand

It has taken over two _____ years for us to make _____ as we know them today. From _____, who used algorithms, to Tim Berners-Lee, who invented the _____, people from all over the _____ have helped to bring us to this point. There are positive and _____ sides to using computers. We need to be _____ about how we use them.

3 What do these words mean?

cipher _____

program _____

algorithm _____

Activity What interests you?

Think about the people you have studied in this unit. Which is the one you have found most interesting? Explain to your teacher what they did, why it is important, and why they are the most interesting to you.

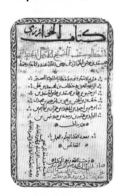
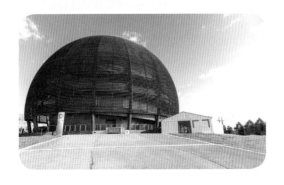
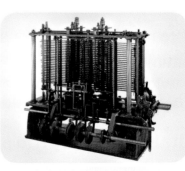

Glossary

algebra a type of mathematics where letters and symbols are used instead of numbers

algorithm a set of rules or instructions for a computer to follow

align to position your text on the page (left, right or centre)

AutoSum a spreadsheet feature that automatically adds the Sum function to a spreadsheet

bar chart a graph that uses oblong bars to compare values

binary representing any number using 0 or 1

cell one box in the spreadsheet grid

cell reference the name of a cell – it is made of the column letter and the row number, for example A1

cipher (also called a code) letters, numbers or symbols used to hide a secret message

composition the way a photograph is designed, for example where the subject is placed in the photograph

copy to make another version of something, so that there are now two of it

copyright when we have made or written something, we usually own it. Anyone who wants to copy and use our creation must ask our permission

crop to make a picture smaller by cutting away some of its edges

cut to remove something, such as a word, so that it is held in another place for a short time

data facts and figures – data can be stored in the computer

digital photograph a photograph made using a camera that records images as computer files

document a text that is created and stored on a computer

event an action that makes a script start running

feedback your opinion of someone's work that will help them improve it

file a place for storing information on the computer

find and replace to look for a word or set of words and put another word or set of words there instead

formula a command that makes the spreadsheet carry out a calculation

function a mathematical process that takes one or more numbers and makes a new number, for example Sum or Average

hierarchical organised in levels

IF statement a computer command that uses a logical test to choose between two possible results

input anything that goes **IN** to the computer, such as typing on the keyboard or clicking the mouse

internet a network of computers around the world

invention something new that has never been made before

logical test a test in a program with a simple Yes/No answer

output anything that comes **OUT** of the computer, such as a screen display or a sound

paste to insert a copy of something

percentage a way of showing a fraction as an amount out of 100, for example $50\% = \frac{1}{2}$

photo shoot a planned event where a photographer takes photographs for a project

pie chart a graph that shows number values as slices of a circle

program a set of instructions that tell a computer to carry out a task

reference to say where we found work that we have copied and used in our own work

responsible looking after ourselves and other people and things

run to carry out a program on the computer

script instructions that control the actions of a sprite

search to look for something

search engine a computer program that searches the internet for information

search results the links that appear when you do a search using a search engine

search term the words you type into a search engine to look for web pages about a particular topic

segment one slice of a pie chart

shared something that a group of people can access or use

sprite an image on the screen that you control with a computer program

stage the area of the screen where you will see the sprite carry out its actions (in Scratch)

storyboard a simple drawing that shows the order of photos to tell a story – it also shows what should be in each photo

subject the main thing you want to show in a photograph

sum a function that calculates the total of a group of numbers

tag a short description of a photo – you can use tags to search for the photo later

USB (Universal Serial Bus) a way of connecting a camera or other device to your computer so that you can share photographs and other files between the devices

variable a value stored by the computer – it has a name and the value stored in the variable can change

webquest an online search

workflow a specific sequence of steps in a task